THE FIRST BREATH

The First Breath

*How Modern Medicine Saves
the Most Fragile Lives*

OLIVIA GORDON

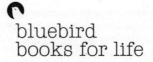

bluebird
books for life

First published 2019 by Bluebird
an imprint of Pan Macmillan
20 New Wharf Road, London N1 9RR
Associated companies throughout the world
www.panmacmillan.com

HB ISBN 978-1-5098-7117-9
TPB ISBN 978-1-5098-7118-6

1 3 5 7 9 8 6 4 2

A CIP catalogue record for this book is available from the British Library.

Typeset in 12.53/16.85 pt Adobe Garamond Pro by Jouve (UK), Milton Keynes
Printed and bound by CPI Group (UK) Ltd, Croydon, CRO 4YY

Visit **www.panmacmillan.com** to read more about all our books
and to buy them. You will also find features, author interviews and
news of any author events, and you can sign up for e-newsletters
so that you're always first to hear about our new releases.

For 'Joel'. I love you infinitely and forever.

And for Lyndall and Siamon Gordon.

When I felt low, my parents were the ones I turned to first, and they were with me whenever I needed any kind of help. I only really understood once I had my own child what extraordinary parents I have. Their love has always been unconditional, as is mine for them.

AUTHOR'S NOTE

Some children's and parents' names, and sometimes identifying details, have been changed to protect privacy, and also to allow people to speak freely.

Some parts of this book were originally published in earlier forms (in the *Guardian*, *The Times*, the *Telegraph*, *Nursing Standard*, the *Daily Mail*, the *Huffington Post* and *Red*), and their reuse is gratefully acknowledged.

Contents

Preface

'Until twenty years ago, children this medically complex
didn't exist. They didn't survive. High-tech medicine
has created a new strain of human beings who require
superhuman care. Society has yet to acknowledge this
reality, especially at a practical level.'

IAN BROWN, THE BOY IN THE MOON BROWN, 2009[1]

This is a story about love and fear: the love and fear a parent
feels for a child who is still unknown; the love and fear doctors
and nurses feel but don't show when they try to save that
child's life. It's a story of bravery: the bravery of pioneering
doctors and nurses who have to risk a child's death to give life;
the bravery of a mother and baby who have no other choice
and who believe they are anything but brave.

This is a story of living through medical history, a history so
recent it happened within my own generation's lifetime. New
fields of medicine built in the last decades of the twentieth
century and the dawn of the twenty-first have saved a generation of children who would not have survived before, whose
first breaths come only thanks to teams of fetal medics and
neonatologists. This medicine has also created a new generation of parents who raise these survivor children.

Almost all the parents I interviewed for this book are people

I have met in the course of my life as a mother of a child with a difference, a 'special' child. If you're not a member of this group, you might not realize how many of us there are these days. Our children don't always have noticeable disabilities, but, at a very young age, they have been through more challenges than many people face in a lifetime. They may be growing up with rare genetic conditions, or may be survivors of fetal surgery, prematurity or congenital organ defects. They may (or may not) have subtle neuropsychiatric differences – autistic spectrum, attention-deficit, sensory processing and/or dyspraxic traits and developmental delays. What they have in common is that they are part of a new group of people whose lives began with an unprecedented level of medical intervention. In many cases they have diagnoses which were impossible to pinpoint until recent years.

As a mother of one such child, without even trying to find others, I meet them everywhere I go. Until the late twentieth century, even when they survived infancy, children growing up with disabilities were often hidden in institutions, educated entirely outside the mainstream, or otherwise excluded from society. Today it's a different story, so I didn't have to search for parents to talk with.

I found myself the mother of a baby whose life was saved by cutting-edge medicine – and this book tells my story, and those of other mothers. Modern science is affecting mothers in the most profound way and I believe it's time to pay more attention to the female experience of medicine. Fathers' experiences are of course just as important as mothers', but this is a book primarily about what it's like to become a mother when pregnancy doesn't go to plan. What it's like to *be* one of the young people of this new generation is yet another story in itself. As is what it's like to have a sick baby without access to the medical privileges of the first world. There are so many stories to tell.

I had an impressionistic, emotional and highly personal understanding of what happened in my own story of motherhood. But I became fascinated by the science and medicine that had touched my family's life so deeply – from histories to principles to practice – and wanted to learn more. I decided to turn my journalist's eye on my own experiences; in effect, to investigate my own case history. What if a patient tried to understand her doctors? Turning from vulnerable patient's mother to writer and reporter would involve a change of relationship with all-powerful doctors, perhaps.

A journalist's job is to investigate and report – to learn from experts. I am a writer who loves science, and I am the mother of a child with a medical condition, not a scientist. My research for this book scratches the surface of multiple complex medical fields. I could spend a lifetime digging just a little deeper and still know next to nothing: the more one knows, the more one realizes how little one knows. I apologize for my ignorance and am immensely grateful to those doctors and scientists who shared their expertise with me. Any mistakes are my own.

1

Abnormality

'Every bump is a mystery . . .'

PROFESSOR ANNA DAVID, FETAL MEDICINE CONSULTANT

One muggy August day in 2015, I sat in a large treatment room at the end of a corridor in central London, watching as consultant obstetrician George Attilakos placed a knife in a kidney dish on a small wheeled table. Together with midwives Ignacio Rosas and Georgina Fox, he laid out everything he needed for the invasive procedure he was about to perform on a woman seventeen weeks pregnant with twins: gauze, syringes, needles, large sterile dressings and plastic and metal tubes. The floor around the bed was covered in paper towels.

At three o'clock, the patient walked in, wearing a hospital gown. Emma was twenty-eight, and, in the world outside, a cheerful, robust office manager and mother of a toddler.

The surgery she was here to have – fetoscopic laser treatment, burning the blood vessels in her placenta to disconnect her twins, who had developed twin-to-twin transfusion syndrome – is one of the more intense procedures the fetal medicine unit of University College Hospital (UCH) undertakes, and is not done lightly.

Emma and her partner Tom, a taxi driver, from north London, had had a complicated pregnancy. At four months, a scan revealed one twin had acrania – the baby was developing without a skull and wouldn't survive after it was born. Emma and Tom were sent here, one of Britain's leading fetal medicine centres, which treat the most problematic pregnancies. Then, on this overcast day, the doctors told them there was a 'time bomb' in Emma's womb.

Blood vessels in the twins' shared placenta were giving one baby too much blood and the other too little, which meant the twin without acrania was likely to die, too. Laser treatment has many risks but gave an 80 per cent chance that the well baby would survive – there was simply no other option. Doctors treat forty cases of twin-to-twin transfusion syndrome each year here, one of only a few hospitals in Britain to do this.

Emma lay on the bed with an absorbent towel tucked into her pants. Naturally a chatty, confident person, she was breathing deeply: 'I'm really nervous.' She was draped from neck to toe, only her belly exposed. The doctor and midwives tried to be reassuring – 'Most women afterwards say it's not as bad as they think,' said Mr Attilakos, gowning up – but Emma radiated anxiety as she was handed a pair of dark glasses to protect her eyes from laser rays. She moaned and sang to herself. Then she sighed: 'I don't want to see anything,' and squeezed her eyes shut.

Georgina said, 'Sweetheart, I know you're scared. You're going to be fine. Nice cup of tea for you afterwards.'

'How many times have you done this before?' Emma asked Mr Attilakos.

'Seventy,' he said.

'Is it tricky for you?'

'No.'

He warned her, though: 'Even if it goes well, you could still miscarry.'

With Tom holding Emma's hand, it was time to start. A local anaesthetic was injected into Emma's belly and Mr Attilakos scanned her using ultrasound, then plunged a needle into her womb, to one side of her belly button. 'Owowowow,' Emma cried. 'It stings.' Georgina held her hand.

Standing at the foot of the bed, observing in my role as a reporter, I thought it looked barbaric. Memories came back from my own similar experience here, five years before, when another specialist, Professor Donald Peebles, pushed a shunt into my unborn baby's thorax to save his life from a deadly condition called hydrops.

I longed to give Emma some words of reassurance, but I couldn't break the concentration and sterile atmosphere surrounding the operation.

*

I'll always remember the ordinariness of the last journey before my own life changed – the feel of the plastic handrails as I calmly sat on the bus, going down Highgate Hill. Later, I found myself wondering how I could not have known that life would never be the same again.

It was a Monday; 4 January 2011. That Christmas, I had been swollen with pregnancy; my mother-in-law seemed amazed by the size of my rock-hard bump for just twenty-seven weeks. We thought I was carrying a big bonny baby. 'He's a little chubster,' my husband Phil laughed.

On Christmas Day, Phil gave me a bottle of eau de parfum. A year later, I would rediscover it, unused. I also wanted a handbag that Christmas – something grown-up, subtle and mature to match the new identity coming my way: 'mother'. I didn't get one, but a few months later I thought about that wish for a handbag and couldn't imagine how I'd have found any use for it or identified with it in the slightest, just as I didn't get any time or desire to wear perfume. Phil gave me a beautiful sewing box – the wooden kind that folds out – but it stood empty on the living room floor for a year. Another gift of several large candles, from our friends Nina and Kris who came to dinner that last New Year's Eve, was, a year on, still wrapped and sitting by our fireplace where I had put it on New Year's Day, planning to start using the candles later that week.

That New Year's Day, Phil and I went to one of our favourite cafes and made a list of things we needed for the nursery and baby. When I found that jokey and innocent list again, a few months later, I could hardly bear to look at it. I'd thought I might buy a breast pump to express occasionally. 'Nappies!!' Phil had written playfully, unthinkingly. A musician – a composer-turned-improviser – and writer who had 'escaped' Sunderland in the north of England for a life of concerts and culture in London, Phil had met me when he was thirty-four and I was twenty-eight. I loved his curly red hair, his nerdy kindness and intellect, and the flattened lilt of a northern accent with which he told jokes. We had both always wanted children. That day we were excited to think our baby would be with us at the end of March. We had no idea that I wouldn't be giving birth in March or even in February; that we wouldn't need to buy and use nappies at home for many more months; that small ordinary things like this, which most parents take for granted, would, for us, be gaping absences.

The Sunday afternoon just after New Year, I fell asleep. I woke to hear Phil on the phone to a friend in New York whose wife was due to give birth in late March, like me. They were comparing how big we were. As I got up, I noticed an odd stitch-like sensation in my twenty-nine-weeks-pregnant belly.

The next morning, I was supposed to go back to my work as a freelance journalist – I had a deadline for Tuesday. But the odd feeling was still there. Just a bug or indigestion, for sure, but I supposed I'd better run it past the midwives. They told me to come in and get assessed. I called Phil away from his desk so we could go to our local north London hospital, the Whittington. It was only a half-hour journey on the bus, and we assumed we'd be sent home within two hours to get on with planning our childbirth classes.

Having miscarried my first pregnancy had made me ultra-anxious this time. Throughout the twenty-nine weeks of this, my second pregnancy, I had been exceedingly cautious, even though I realized my fears were excessive. I hadn't painted my nails, stood near a smoker, eaten forbidden foods – not once. It was as if by worrying constantly and following the recommended guidelines to the letter, I could ward off anything truly bad happening. Pregnancy, I was to discover, has no regard for superstition.

It hadn't been a straightforward six months. I had bled on and off through the first trimester and had several early scans. When the midwife told me: 'Go home and put your feet up,' I was so paranoid about not following her advice to the letter that I was afraid to stand up. Then at our thirteen-week ante-natal screening, we'd had the nuchal translucency test, a scan which measures the fluid at the back of the baby's neck.

3.01 mm is a number I'll never forget. It was the exact width of a black space at the back of our baby's neck, and the fact that it was over 3 mm, I was told, could be a sign it had Down's syndrome, or another chromosomal condition. Like many, I had accepted the screening test offered to me without much thought, assuming that the result would be normal. I'd had weeks of bleeding and early scans, but the solemn reaction of the sonographer when she measured the fluid under the skin of our child's neck and found it just a little too much was the first official red flag Phil and I had that this pregnancy wasn't typical.

I'd hit Google and found a world of pregnant women panicking about their numbers. My baby's result was just above the borderline, but along with stories from women who had had high numbers and 'normal' babies, I read many stories of pregnancies with measurements like ours where the fetuses were found to have abnormalities and terminated. It seemed that even being 0.1 mm over the 3 mm cut-off point was cause for concern. Never before in my life had a minute number held such significance. I looked at the scan photo again and again, at that black space deemed just a little too big, wondering how such a small thing could be pinpointed accurately.

Together, the nuchal and blood test results gave every woman a ratio, the chance of her baby having one of the commonest chromosomal syndromes: Down's, Edwards' or Patau's. I read that a high nuchal translucency was also associated with heart conditions and one or two other genetic syndromes – it all sounded obscure and unlikely; a world away. My blood test results turned out unremarkable, so my given chance of a child with a chromosomal condition was only one in several hundred, a relatively high ratio but nothing compared to the women whose ratios were one in three or one in twenty.

For the first time since schoolgirl maths lessons, I thought about probability. Most of the women with high ratios did have invasive tests – chorionic villus sampling (CVS) or amniocentesis – and after anxious posts debating what a chance of one in thirty or one in ten really meant, they returned to the online forums to broadcast their relief – 'Everything's normal, thank God' – and to be congratulated. We would not have considered ending the pregnancy unless our child had a condition incompatible with life and we chose not to undergo the risk of invasive tests.

Although there was the occasional mention online of a diagnosis with Patau's or Edwards', almost always followed by a termination because these trisomies are generally considered incompatible with life long after birth, most of the talk – and anxiety – surrounded the possibility of having a baby with the far more common Down's syndrome. A few voices crept in saying Down's wasn't something to fear, but they were drowned out by other women reassuring the worried: 'I had a high risk and my baby didn't have Down's – he's a gorgeous, healthy baby.'

Noting how frightened other pregnant women were of Down's, and the NHS offering screening for it to all pregnant women, it was hard not to become frightened, too.

At twenty weeks, after extra scans, including a fetal echocardiogram to examine our baby's heart, we were told he was a boy and everything was 'beautiful'. The cardiologist said, 'Go away and enjoy the rest of your pregnancy.'

At last, I finally felt relatively safe. Every time we had been for scans before, we'd been terrified something was wrong, and rushed to the hospital by Tube. This early day of a new year, it was different. We were in the third trimester; everything was 'beautiful'. So we took the bus, as if to underline that we were in a safe new place now.

When we got to triage, where I was examined on a row of couches next to two other pregnant women, the midwives couldn't find anything wrong, apart from the fact their tape measures suggested I was around thirty-five weeks pregnant rather than twenty-nine. But then, it's so easy to mis-measure with a tape measure. They wondered if I might have placental abruption – a separation of the placenta from the uterus – and decided to keep me in overnight. It was my first ever night on a hospital ward, lying in my little curtained cubicle among twenty other pregnant women, and I couldn't sleep. I emailed my editor to say I'd be back the next day.

The next day, Tuesday, I was told I could go home as soon as they'd scanned me. As we walked down the corridor towards the ultrasound room, I couldn't wait to see our baby again. How lucky to get an extra scan at such a late stage. Phil and I held hands.

I lay there being scanned and I saw the baby on the screen and I was happy and saying, 'Oh wow! He's moving! Look at those legs!' And then I noticed the sonographer was very quiet.

Finally, she said something.

'Er – it looks like there's a lot of amniotic fluid.'

'Oh,' we said. It didn't sound too bad. But it did explain why I hadn't felt much movement the last few hours.

Then she continued, 'These are pleural effusions – fluid around the lungs – and it looks like there's fluid under the scalp.'

'What does that mean?' I asked.

She paused awkwardly.

I asked, 'Is this serious?'

All this time, I'd been worrying about something going wrong, and now it seemed it actually was. This wasn't supposed to happen.

'I'm sorry. I'm not allowed to go into any detail,' she said, her voice withdrawn. There was no smile. 'You'll have to see the consultant.'

'But is it a bad thing?' I asked.

'I'm afraid it's not great news,' she replied, poker-faced.

It was from that moment that everything changed.

We were taken back to the ward, where we waited and

waited for a doctor to come. Night fell; my mother's chicken casserole, waiting at home, grew cold.

A young, anxious-looking junior doctor finally came to my cubicle and pulled the curtain closed. Our baby, he explained, had a rare condition called hydrops fetalis, affecting around one in 3,000 pregnancies, many of which, associated with conditions like Edwards' syndrome or toxoplasmosis, usually end spontaneously, sooner or later during pregnancy. For whatever reason, the body's lymphatic, or drainage, system fails. Our baby was breathing in amniotic fluid but not processing it; it was building up within both of us, crushing his lungs, restricting his growth and filling my womb, putting him at risk of premature birth.

'What's going to happen to him?' I dared to ask. 'What is his chance of living?'

'I can't give you a chance,' the doctor said.

Did he mean there was no chance at all? I couldn't ask this question.

The doctor stumbled over his words, as if he was unsure. He kept saying a consultant would come to see me and would explain everything properly.

From the cubicle next to me, separated by a floaty curtain, I could hear a doctor talking to a mother about her gestational diabetes. She was crying. I was shocked to find myself feeling, of all things, envy. I wished I was having a 'typical' pregnancy hospital conversation.

I asked to be moved from the ward with the other pregnant women. I was sent to the labour ward. Not because I was about to give birth imminently, but so I could have a room of my own. It was much more comfortable than the antenatal ward, although all night I heard the women in labour, doing their thing, screaming, it seemed to me, in a sort of blithe innocence.

New fathers lugged car seats around, looking proud and important. Outside the toilet, one woman dripped pools of bright red blood on the linoleum. I no longer identified with these people. I wouldn't have antenatal care or give birth at this hospital. I was to be transferred to University College Hospital, where there was a specialist fetal medicine unit for pregnancies like mine, where the baby was in trouble.

The Irish midwife was kind, coming in to take my vital signs every few hours. My mother stayed by my side all night. Sometime around 2 a.m., I drifted. Then at eight in the morning, an obstetric consultant came to see me. Sometimes, a gesture of caring when you're really scared in hospital can actually be frightening. When a senior doctor comes to see you – having put you first on his list – with compassion in his eyes and reaches out as he leaves to pat you on the shoulder and says, 'You're being very strong,' you know this is bad. As the day went on, and we were scanned again, we saw the most senior obstetricians the hospital had to offer.

I wasn't being strong; I was just living through this. The first scan had been on Tuesday afternoon; thanks to the NHS, at noon on Friday we, my parents and Phil's mother stepped through the doors of UCH, a glass-walled modern hospital in the centre of London. On the first floor of the obstetric wing, we followed signs which diverted us from the general antenatal care area to a set of closed doors marked Fetal Medicine Unit. I sanitized my hands carefully at the dispenser and called my family back to sanitize theirs, too. There were only a few other pregnant women in the waiting room – two simple rows of chairs and a water dispenser – all of us sitting quietly. No one was being called; every so often a doctor or midwife in blue scrubs walked past. We waited for forty-five minutes, watching the clock ticking. A notice on the wall read: 'Please be aware you may have a long waiting time due to the nature of the Fetal Medicine Unit'.

Then a door opened and a sensible, friendly-looking mid-wife with straight brown hair and glasses called my name. Phil and I – and my father, a doctor himself – were ushered through the door into an ultrasound suite. There, tall and patrician Professor Donald Peebles shook our hands and told us that hydrops was, frankly, not an everyday problem.

I'd Googled him and found out that he was the hospital's head of research in maternal and fetal medicine and had two grown-up daughters. He divided his time between research into the physiology of unborn babies and clinical practice, in fetal medicine and also as an obstetrician. Professor Peebles would one day tell me that fetal medicine 'poses a completely different set of ethical challenges because there are two patients – mum and fetus. Sometimes they're at odds. And although the focus is on the baby, all the interaction is with the mother.' For now, I was one such mother. The prof was like his online picture – a distinguished-looking man in a suit, smiling reassuringly but, more than anything, cool and matter-of-fact. Doctors working with ill babies can't appear sentimental, I was to learn. Their job is to give the patient the facts, even if they are bad.

I had also Googled hydrops and the word 'fatal' had leaped into my vision again and again; there was line after line and page after page of that word. Most babies, I'd read, die in the womb or don't live long after a premature birth. Phil refused to look at my pages of Google searches and medical journal write-ups about dead hydropic fetuses. He believed that every-thing would be all right. But I'd kept Googling, unable to look away from the computer screen.

Now I lay on the couch while Professor Peebles scanned me using a state-of-the-art ultrasound machine. I hoped he would find things weren't so bad, but the fluid all around our baby and inside his scalp and chest was still there and, if anything, was getting worse. Professor Peebles and the midwife looked serious. Our only potential treatment, Peebles told us, was an emergency invasive procedure – draining the excess fluid from the baby and womb, and inserting a plastic 'shunt', a coiled plastic drainage tube, halfway into the baby's chest wall, to drain more fluid from his chest into my amniotic sac.

The shunt treatment, he said, was the only treatment. He had done it before, but not that often – the unit only did this procedure five times a year, since hydrops is rare. The longer we left it, the less chance our baby had. It had to go ahead right now. The shunt could well fail; the risks were many.

No one could tell us why this was happening. Hydrops often develops with no known cause or could be connected to anything from genetic conditions to infections. The unit would do every test available. It was gently mentioned that we had the right to abort this pregnancy if the situation deteriorated. But my thoughts gathered on a different fate: if the baby didn't respond to the fetal procedure and died of hydrops, I would give birth to a stillborn.

Phil and I signed the consent form for the operation and my father returned to the waiting room to update the prospective grandmothers, who were in a state of controlled anxiety. 'We've contacted the neonatal unit and they have a cot ready – there's a one in three chance you'll go into premature labour,' said Peebles.

I'd never seen a neonatal unit. Phil didn't even know what a neonatal unit was. We had no idea what would go on there. It was hard to imagine the creature under my skin as a living baby, but it was reassuring to hear that if he did come early, the doctors thought they could treat him. He must have some chance, then.

I asked to go to the ladies' while Peebles and the junior doctor and nurse prepared for the procedure. There, I looked in the mirror and steeled myself. 'Is this happening?' I asked. 'Am I going to let them cut into my unborn baby in five minutes?' My answer to myself was 'Yes.' I took a deep breath.

Back in the darkened scanning room, I lay on the examination couch with my belly and baby exposed and vulnerable. They swabbed cold antiseptic onto my abdomen and injected local anaesthetic. At this point I turned my head to the right so I couldn't see any more. Phil sat on my left, holding my hand. The brown-haired nurse, whose name was Nicky, was so gentle, holding my feet and asking, 'Are you all right?' Peebles was going to watch his operation on the ultrasound screen so he could see what he was doing. Phil watched the screen. I didn't want to close my eyes but I stared at the edge of the room.

First Peebles inserted a needle through my abdomen into one side of my womb and drained out – I later saw – several litre bottles of amniotic fluid. There was so much that it splashed into his shoes, making him shout almost comically in surprise. The pressure in my belly relieved, and the baby one step safer, he then moved on to what the doctors called 'shunting'.

Phil later described to me what he had seen. Peebles watched the screen intently as he stood poised over a point on the other side of my bump, holding a cannula (tube) mounted on a sharp, thick needle. At an instant when our baby moved to one side of the womb and grew still, Peebles called 'Now!' and plunged the cannula very quickly into my belly, into my womb, into our baby's chest. I felt the visceral deep force of this plunge and cried out. It was as if Peebles was playing a video game or taking a pot shot at a coconut. Basic.

The 'oooh' groans I was making came instinctively and sounded animal-like. It wasn't so much pain as surprise and strangeness for our unexpecting baby. It felt wrong; the antithesis of every effort I'd made to keep my baby safe in pregnancy.

There was a pause and then everyone breathed with relief as our baby moved again. Peebles pushed the 'shunt' – a drainage tube – into the cannula, then pulled out the cannula and needle. The shunt seemed to be in place, halfway into the baby's chest and halfway out, though it was hard for Peebles to be sure. The whole procedure had taken half an hour.

The midwife gave me a womb relaxant to reduce the chance of labour and monitored the baby. I was his only link with the world and so I pressed a button every time I felt him move.

Over the next ten days at home, I tried to move as little as possible to avoid miscarrying, and I Googled, reading stories of mothers who had lost child after child to unexplained hydrops. That word, which I had never heard before, and which no one in my non-medical world knew, and which was mentioned in absolutely none of my fifteen pregnancy manuals, was like a portal to a dark new world. I strung together enough words for that article I'd been on deadline for, then stopped work. I lay in the bath and couldn't stop thinking about what I was sure was going to happen, which was that my baby would die in the womb and I would have to give birth to him . . . and that then I would never be able to have another baby; every pregnancy would end in hydrops. From my bedside window, I watched the neighbours in our frosty suburban street coming in and out of their houses with their children; mothers wheeling prams. In my mind, I wasn't properly pregnant any more; I wasn't one of them. I felt an odd embarrassment at my failure to have a healthy baby.

I couldn't sleep and asked my parents to stay day and night. Late one night I crawled into my mother's arms and she held me like a baby. I thought only my husband and family could see me like this; I only group-emailed my friends to let them know what was happening. But Grace, my old schoolfriend since the age of eleven, was determined to speak to me. So, from a Goan beach where she was beginning a six-month career break from her job as a PA, she insisted Phil put me on the phone.

'I'm going to fly home,' she said as she waded in the sea. 'I want to be with you. Call me any time of the night.'

'Oh, it's not necessary,' I replied automatically.

I don't believe in God, but I prayed for half-hours at a time – sometimes to God or Jesus (because he loved children), sometimes to my baby himself, sometimes to a vague idea of some god of motherhood who might save him. I lay on my bed and murmured these prayers to my baby; I hoped he was somehow listening.

One especially dark Sunday afternoon, I found myself driving to my local synagogue in suburban north London. I'd never been before; it was an anonymous, brutalist building in a row of semi-detached houses. I could see the rabbi and a group of people having a small gathering inside. I knocked on the door until someone heard me, and was ushered in, feeling surreal and biblical, with my swollen pregnant belly.

I told my story to the bemused rabbi. 'I know I've never been here before,' I said, 'and I'm not religious, but would you pray for my baby?'

'Of course,' he said. We lit a candle and prayed.

On Tuesday my phone rang. 'The chromosomal result is normal,' the fetal unit midwife had to repeat again and again because I needed endless reassurance. Our baby didn't have a chromosomal abnormality; this wasn't Edwards', Patau's or Down's syndrome. Tests for serious viral infections – toxoplasmosis and parvovirus – were also negative. More tests could be done at birth, but for now, the cause of the hydrops remained 'unknown'. In one way, that was good – nothing else had been found. In another way, it was bad – unexplained hydrops can repeat in future pregnancies, and in my mind I was already thinking about my lack of ability to have any children. I started Googling adoption.

I also phoned the Down's Syndrome Association and selected the option to make a donation. 'That's very kind of you,' said the woman who processed it. 'May I take your name?'

'Thank you, but I'd like to be anonymous,' I said.

There was a pause before she politely said: 'Oh . . . Well, yes, that's fine.' I knew she was wondering who the hell I was. Little did this nice woman from the charity imagine, I thought, that she was talking to a heavily pregnant woman moved by guilty relief.

A few days after the shunt treatment, Phil and I returned for more scans with the director of the fetal medicine unit, Pranav Pandya, a slim, smiley man I imagined playing carefree games of tennis or yachting in his spare time. We had hoped the fluid in our baby's chest, which appeared on the scan as two black pools – dark and unknown – would have shrunk. We might need to be 'shunted' again if the shunt had ended up totally inside or outside our son's chest rather than halfway in, though of course each operation carried greater risk. And so it turned out – the shunt had ended up lodged all the way in our baby's chest, and so could not drain the amniotic fluid collecting there. But for the moment, Mr Pandya told us in his reassuringly breezy manner, the overall volume of fluid was much better.[†]

'When you first came in, your baby's chances of survival were 50–50,' Pandya said at a scan a week after our shunt, 'but now it's gone up to 80 per cent and I'd even say now it's at 90.' Every day the baby could stay inside me now, without needing shunting again, the better.

Three days later, I felt the pressure in my stomach return and I started bleeding. The initial shunt operation had saved my son's life for another few weeks in the womb, but no longer.

Getting through the fetal medicine unit is only the first hurdle for a very sick baby. The worst for our son Joel – and for me – was still to come, during our time in neonatal care. Joel's recovery was to be long and complex. During his first five months as an inpatient, he would be cared for by more than a hundred specialist doctors and nurses in three different hospitals. We were just another family to them, but to us, they were gods.

*

Years passed but I found I couldn't leave that hospital experience behind. It haunted me, as a mother. And I had good reason to believe it haunted my son on some level, too.

I realized I was a member of an increasing band of parents whose children would not have survived, could not have been treated, if born thirty, twenty or even ten years before. Modern medicine had saved our children; we had our 'miracle babies', but beyond the sentimental 'little warrior' clichés, we

[†] In the UK, senior surgeons (including obstetricians and gynaecologists) often use the title Mr or Miss (or Ms/Mrs) instead of Dr.

faced a reality of children with complex needs and our own uncharted emotions, after our bizarre initiation into parenthood. Saving our children was uncharted territory for the medical staff, too.

A fetus in the womb was unreachable and a mystery to previous generations; today doctors can diagnose illness from the early weeks of pregnancy (and even before implantation) and are saving babies' lives with operations in utero, and intensive care and surgery after birth. My child is one of this new generation. No one knows quite what their lives will be like.

I eventually worked out that I had been lucky, as the shell-shocked mother of a critically ill baby, to live just half an hour away from one of the world's leading centres for fetal medicine, a young, highly specialized and dynamic field of medicine which is saving the lives of unborn babies who aren't growing normally, who will need operations after birth, or with a huge range of disorders. The unit at UCH is one of around seven leading fetal medicine centres in England offering therapies like laser surgery for twin-to-twin transfusion syndrome.[1] Doctors at my hospital, I would later discover, were among the first in the world to treat fetuses and neonates, and in 2018 they became the first in Britain to offer open fetal surgery – in which surgeons open the womb, operate on the fetus, then seal the baby back into the womb for the pregnancy to (hopefully) continue. Parents are referred from hospitals all over the country.

After my son was well, I wanted to go back and see the fetal medicine and neonatal units again, and I wished I could dare to ask the doctors what it had been like for them. I wanted to keep in touch with our doctors. How could I not? They had saved our child's life. When our baby finally came out of hospital, we sent them thank-you cookies; at Christmas we sent cards we hoped they would display along with all the others on the unit walls, with photos of our own 'miracle baby'. Every now and then, Phil or I sent an email with a photo of Joel to Mr Pandya, or Dr Meek at the neonatal unit. They always replied genially, signing their names as Pran and Judith, but I could still only think of them as Mr Pandya and Dr Meek, mysterious heroic figures. During our time in neonatal care, Dr Meek, in particular, had a way of appearing in the room almost magically, like a fairy godmother materializing in a puff of smoke, just when she was most needed.

I wasn't alone in wanting to revisit the units, perinatal hospital psychologist Dr Claudia De Campos mentioned when I interviewed her for a newspaper. Many former patients like to go back – it's a form of catharsis, of digesting a surreal, sudden past experience. (Others, she said, never want to set foot in the hospital again.) Anyway, when, around a year after Joel came home, I tried to go back to UCH to visit our son's past doctors, the astringent hospital smell and the sight of linoleum corridors and hand-sanitizer dispensers made me feel dizzy, and I turned back at the door.

I was haunted as a journalist, too. As a patient, I used to sit in the waiting room and look at the other pregnant women, some smiley, others tearful. I watched as they were ushered behind the closed doors of the consulting rooms and wondered what was going on in there. Again and again, on hearing my own son's shunting story, people told me they had no idea such procedures were possible, let alone being done. I wanted to know what it was like for other mothers and babies, the first generation for whom life before birth has been highly medicalized, and for these doctors who hold not only life and death but also the possibility of birth in their hands. I needed to explore the strange relationship which grows up between the doctor and the family in such circumstances – the professional gap between doctor and patient at odds with the intense personal intimacy of treating that most precious thing, a mother's unborn child.

My fascination with fetal and neonatal medicine grew as time passed and the rawness of my own experience damped down. As a journalist, I found myself choosing to write about my own experience and those of others in newspapers and online; interviewing clinicians; following research. Finally, despite my butterflies, I put my queasiness aside and walked back through the unit's doors as a writer, granted unprecedented access to sit in on dozens of consultations behind closed doors to observe and report on procedures like my own. I felt privileged and emotional to be back with all the staff: Nicky, the calm midwife who had held my hand when I was terrified; cool, collected Peebles; and the upbeat force of nature Mr Pandya himself.

I'd grown up the daughter of an Oxford research scientist and doctor, one who studied the immunology of cells. I'd played Consequences on the back of abstruse scientific papers, but never done Biology GCSE. Instead I grew up wanting to be a writer. My father, the kindest man in the world, only ever allowed the slightest frustration to show when I couldn't grasp some basic maths or physics homework. And now I was a mother of a medical curiosity. That gave me a certain worth in doctors' eyes. But I wanted to cross the line and talk to medical people on their own terms. Although this time I was there as a writer – a professional – not a patient, I still felt nervous. I was sure the doctors remembered my own case as utterly insignificant; after all, they see hundreds of women with critically ill babies every year. I wondered if they thought I was weird for wanting to stay in touch.

And even as Mr Pandya – the friendliest of consultants – hugged me and welcomed me and asked after Joel, there was something about the past relationship between us as doctor and patient that I couldn't quite bridge. I wondered if he felt it too. Patients don't usually go back as reporters. As a journalist trying to research the medical science behind my own experiences, I felt intimidated at the very idea of approaching doctors and scientists to speak to me as some sort of equal; a constant fear that they would raise their eyebrows at my ignorance and tell me I'd written up their work completely wrongly. Or that they'd feel I was after their trade secrets – the inner workings of the hospital, the private backstage protocols that patients, like the audience of a play or the customers of a business, aren't meant to see.

*

That stifling August day in the treatment room, on the surface of Emma's belly, I saw a drop of blood seep out around the needle. Mr Attilakos cut into her stomach with a knife. 'This is the bit that will hurt a little,' he said. The local anaesthetic numbs the skin and the tissue beneath, but sometimes the mother still feels pain from this procedure. He fed a long tube attached to both a laser and a camera down into the needle in Emma's womb, and as he repeatedly jabbed, she shouted: 'Ow, oh fuck, it really hurts.'

'Stay still!' he implored her.

Tom was quietly crying.

'I feel faint,' Emma said. She was burning hot; Georgina fanned her with a cardboard sick basin.

Mr Attilakos was watching the camera's view intently on a large screen. He was looking at the placenta with its lethal shared blood vessels connecting the babies, and he fired on each blood vessel with the laser. On the screen he could see a light flash with each zap, and the tissue evaporating in puffs of smoke as red vessels burned to white. The camera moved slightly and we saw a baby's hand in its silken webbing.

'Try to breathe less deeply,' Mr Attilakos urged Emma. 'When you do a deep breath, it moves everything.' He added: 'You may feel popping; it's a bit alarming.'

'I can feel it in my throat,' Emma said, but Mr Attilakos thought that was sheer anxiety. Georgina tried to lighten the tension: 'These sick bowls come in handy for all sorts of things.'

After forty minutes of laser zapping, they drained nearly a litre of excess amniotic fluid from Emma using the tube in her belly – it would also be checked for chromosomal abnormalities. Mr Attilakos's hands were dripping with amniotic fluid as he pulled the tube out sharply and joked, 'After this you mustn't do any housework for three months!'

The relief that it was over was palpable. Emma and Tom hugged and kissed as they slowly walked to the recovery room. Tomorrow they were to have another scan. 'It's your worst nightmare,' Emma told me. 'You never think this is going to happen to you. We've channelled all our hopes into our well baby.'

The doctors, I saw, felt their pain, and hope, too. Everyone who works at the fetal medicine unit is passionately committed to saving pregnancies – from the team of consultants to the specialist midwives, researchers and receptionists.

Over a few days observing, I watched nervous couples stream into the fetal medicine unit. Sometimes siblings come too, and it is odd to see children, even though children are what this unit is all about, because the world of fetal medicine is a world of black and white scans. As one fetal medicine consultant here, Professor Anna David, put it to me: 'Scanning is like meeting a new person each time – every bump is a mystery and you're like Sherlock Holmes trying to find out what's wrong.'

One average day in the unit started with a twenty-eight-week termination for lethal skeletal dysplasia – a small chest that would leave the baby unable to breathe. 'You just have to do it,' the doctor told me beforehand. 'I don't like to do it but it's far worse for the patient.' The same morning, there was good news for a couple with twins suspected of having cytomegalovirus (a common virus which can cause great damage in pregnancy). Their scan was normal, and Mr Pandya felt the blood test that flagged up the virus was probably a false positive, though they would have further tests. 'I think this is good news – and we really know what we're doing,' he assured the parents as they cried with relief.

Then there was dark news again – a twenty-four-weeker with congenital diaphragmatic hernia: the abdominal organs in the chest, compressing the unformed lungs. Before the mother, accompanied by grandmother-to-be, came in, Dr Fred Ushakov, another leading doctor in the unit, said: 'This is serious. There's a one in three chance the baby will die; more in this case.' The mother, a twenty-five-year-old having her first baby, walked in smiling and despite Mr Pandya explaining after their scan that the baby had a 50–50 chance and gently touching her arm, they left laughing and upbeat. 'Glass half-full,' the grandmother said.

After the door closed behind them, Mr Pandya said, compassionately, 'Tough . . . she was naive, she has no idea. It didn't seem to me she completely comprehended.' Hilary Hewitt, the midwife attending, added: 'Some parents are completely risk-averse; others are blindly optimistic. Others have: "God will get us through". You just have to lay the evidence in front of them.'

Another midwife rushed out to the waiting area where a man was kicking up a fuss about the waiting time. 'Sometimes people can be angry,' Hilary said. 'It's just stress.' Parents come to the business of bad news in different ways, Pran told me. For him, the human interaction in fetal medicine – managing the families through the maze and empathizing with how they feel – was what made him love going to work on a Monday morning.

There were women having reassurance scans after previous pregnancies went wrong; a fetus with sickle-cell anaemia; another whose blood group was incompatible with its mother; conjoined twins; babies with various heart conditions. Some patients came in smiling and shaking hands; others were withdrawn and taciturn.

The decisions the doctors made for parents and babies at such critical moments were difficult. Sarah and Peter, in their thirties, had been coming to the unit every week after their twenty-week scan showed the baby wasn't growing. I listened to senior fetal medicine and neonatal consultants privately discussing this tiny baby. He was twenty-six weeks old and weighed 500g, which made him just viable, but, Peebles sighed, 'It's not good.' Last week the doctors thought he couldn't be saved, but now he had gained this crucial bit of weight, there was some hope. Then again, Peebles had spotted the baby had ascites: worrying fluid around the abdomen, collecting because his heart was struggling.

In the staff room, the doctors and midwives spent a long time deciding what to say to the couple. Finally, neonatologist Sian Harding brought the parents into a quiet room and carefully told them: 'The baby's condition is deteriorating . . .

things may well get worse. If we wait, there's quite a high risk your baby could die in the next few days.'

Sarah and Peter were calm in the way people are in a crisis, speaking through adrenaline. Sarah said stoically, 'Yeah, sure, OK,' as Dr Harding explained that the best option, in her view, was to deliver the baby in the next few days. His chance of survival, then, would be 30 per cent and his chance of life-long disability would be 50–50. Peter said: 'I'm quite worried, to be honest.' Dr Harding replied, in a sensitively measured, neutral tone, that his response was appropriate. Sarah said: 'I'm a more positive person,' and managed a laugh – she was trying to be strong.

I saw several women referred by local hospitals who had been told their babies had a low chance of surviving. Here, they were expertly scanned for the first time and reassured things were not so bad after all. The doctors understood how upset couples can be during scans for anomalies and murmured comfort: 'The heart is beautiful,' Mr Pandya told a mother whose baby had pleural effusions, the same potentially lethal fluid around the lungs which my son had had. Pandya, I saw, was simply brilliant at assessing, making decisions and explaining situations to parents, despite the prognosis of fetal medicine cases being especially hard to judge. 'I'm very confident your baby's going to be fine,' he told the couple. Pandya told me: 'Things are often unclear. A good consultant is just someone who is good at guessing.' He was right. Non-medical people, especially those of us who have studied and worked in the arts, tend to have a naive idea that medicine is an exact science. But a little exposure to medicine had taught Phil and me that it is quite the opposite: vague. And of all areas of medicine, the stakes of fetal medicine – saving a whole life which hasn't even begun, in the body of another living being – are arguably the highest.

I left the fetal medicine unit that week feeling as if I had experienced space travel for the first time. It had been eerie to come so close to death before birth – but I was humbled by medicine's triumph in offering life, at least to some, where there was almost no hope.

Later, I asked Mr Pandya about the outcome for Emma and Tom. One of their twins had acrania and had no hope of living. It was to save the other baby's life that they had undergone the laser surgery for twin-to-twin transfusion syndrome. But this twin also didn't survive, in the end.

Pandya had remarked to me in the unit one morning, 'When the outcome isn't good, it's life-changing for the family, but for the team involved, it's significant too. You get to know them, and to see the parent holding the baby as it's about to die is devastating. You question whether you did the right thing.' The thank-you cards he and his colleagues get after even these terrible experiences mean everything.

This amiable doctor, I learned, wasn't the carefree sportsman I had once imagined him to be when I was his patient. He and his wife had been fetal medicine patients too, when they went through two pregnancies which he described to me as 'harrowing'. He was a father who felt deeply for patients in dire circumstances.

As for me, it's strange to know that my child would not have lived if he had not been born here and now, in a first-rate hospital with access to the latest, greatest technology in modern science. Joel would have had no chance of survival had he been born before the modern era. In one early neonatology textbook, published in 1945, hydrops fetalis was simply described as a condition 'incompatible with life . . . the infant is either still-born or dies shortly after birth'.[2] Even if Joel had been conceived in the year I was born, 1978, he would still have died a fetus, his lungs crushed by amniotic fluid.

Yet here I am writing this, the mother of a cuddly, whimsical little chatterbox who asks for sausages for dinner every day and can't quite decide which snake he prefers, the boomslang or the inland taipan.

I decided to find out how, exactly, modern medicine got my son here.

2

High-Risk Case

'The fetus as a patient is truly a miracle. And it seems that
our first crude attempts at fetal treatment are only tinkering
at the edge of this miracle. It has been our great privilege to
be tinkerers. We have been lucky enough to reach out and
occasionally touch this miracle.'

MICHAEL HARRISON, THE 'FATHER' OF FETAL SURGERY[1]

In a quiet room at the Children's Hospital of Philadelphia
(CHOP), Dan Seabold, a scrub nurse, waited anxiously for
news. He worked assisting in operating theatres, but now he
found himself on the other side; a patient, of sorts. His twenty-
five-weeks pregnant wife Kelly was unconscious in the
operating theatre at America's leading fetal medicine centre,
the hospital's surgeon-in-chief Dr N. Scott Adzick cutting
into her womb to operate on the unborn baby.

The Seabolds flew from their home in Cleveland to Philadelphia for the surgery in 2015. Baby Maeve's heart was
shutting down as a result of a gigantic sacrococcygeal teratoma
(SCT) discovered at the twenty-week scan; a tumour at the
base of her tailbone. The rich blood flow into the tumour was
causing hydrops, straining the capabilities of the tiny fetal
heart. And Kelly was also sick, with a condition called maternal mirror syndrome – her body was taking on symptoms

from the sick fetus's heart failure; her body's tissues were accumulating excess fluid. The situation was critical, but there was one chance to save Maeve's life: radical open fetal surgery, first successfully performed for SCT in 1997, by Dr Adzick. At the time of writing, an operation on a fetus with SCT has only been tried ten times since, with seven survivors.

The surgery would, ideally, go like this. Dr Adzick would make an incision in Kelly's uterus under general anaesthetic, cut out the tumour, which was nearly the same size as the fetus, stabilize the baby and close the baby back in the uterus. Performing an experimental surgery like this, the risks were monumental. There were three ways the doctors thought the operation could turn out. The baby could recover and the pregnancy could continue under close scrutiny with Kelly on bed rest – after surgery, Kelly would be brought back to this intensive care room, where she would be bathed with ice water to stop her overheating because she was to be given so much magnesium sulphate to help prevent uterine contractions which could lead to premature birth after surgery. But most likely, being so young and sick, the baby would not tolerate surgery and die. Or the baby and the mother could fall ill within a few days after the operation, and the child would have to be delivered extremely premature, and only have a fighting chance of survival. Kelly had been wheeled to surgery pregnant; no one knew if she would still be pregnant when she came back.

At 9.30 a.m., two hours after Kelly had gone to theatre, around the time Dan was tensely pacing, expecting her to return, a neonatologist came into the room. The tumour had been removed – but Maeve was not doing well.

When Dr Adzick had opened the uterus, the amniotic fluid was the colour of port wine; it was full of blood. He had a moment to register that the tumour must have ruptured just before the start of surgery. And then, the baby's heart stopped.

The doctors gave Maeve emergency medicine through the umbilical vein to resuscitate her. Dr Adzick even did fetal chest compressions with his finger. Maeve came back.

But then, while he was cutting the tumour away from her, Maeve went into cardiac arrest again ('which was very inconvenient,' Adzick later told me in his characteristically laconic style). They managed, again, to resuscitate her.

Kelly's uterus had contracted during the operation and there wasn't much space for Maeve to be placed back inside. Her head was already in, and eventually Adzick managed to relax the uterus enough to start to get her bottom half back inside.

It was then that Maeve had a third cardiac arrest ('somewhat discouraging', as Adzick put it to me). She was extraordinarily anaemic; they gave her a blood transfusion, medication, and her heart finally restarted after nearly ten minutes of resuscitation. But getting Maeve back into the uterus continued to be extremely tricky. Adzick really didn't know if it would be possible or not.

The neonatologist had come to ask Dan what he would like them to do. They might have to deliver Maeve, but her chance of surviving would be minimal at best and even then, she could be brain damaged. But it seemed even less likely that they would get Maeve back in the womb with a heartbeat. Dan gave his consent to deliver Maeve.

Dan, together with Kelly's parents, watched, mute, as the nurse dismantled the equipment around the bed waiting for Kelly. They wouldn't need all this stuff if she wasn't going to be pregnant.

At 10.45, the nurse returned to the room. She began hurriedly setting the equipment back up. 'Why are you doing this?' Dan asked. That was when the nurse apologized for her silence and explained. Adzick had tried – just one last time – to place Maeve back in the uterus, having plastered the inside of the uterine membranes and wall with Teflon felt to strengthen it. And he had done it; she was back in, her heart still beating. Kelly was still pregnant. Dan was overwhelmed with emotion.

Dr Adzick walked into the room. He appeared deep in thought, even slightly stunned. 'Well, that sure wasn't easy,' Dr Adzick said. The normally urbane, confident surgeon recounted his repeated attempts to resuscitate Maeve and how he'd recalled his early career experiments on animals to find a way to bring Maeve back. He later told the couple this was one of the most difficult operations he had ever performed. When Kelly and Dan recounted this story to me of the most challenging day of their lives, Maeve was two years old – and thriving.

I asked Dr Adzick what the operation was like from his perspective. 'You're British,' he said. 'So, Churchill . . . Never give in, right?'

*

Until recently, babies with congenital defects would often die in the womb or be born severely disabled.[†] Babies as ill as Maeve – and my son – would still have no chance of life today, had it not been for an outlandish and controversial idea

† Congenital defects are often called 'birth defects', but as the guru of fetal medicine Michael Harrison has pointed out: 'we now realise that these are not "birth defects"; they are defects that become manifest at birth, but have a long and interesting history before birth.' Michael Harrison, *Atlas of Fetal Surgery*, Chapman & Hall, 1996, p5.

striking a trainee paediatric surgeon in the 1970s[2] – a possible way to give life and health to those doomed babies.

Michael Harrison, born the son of a country doctor in the Pacific Northwest in 1944, had graduated cum laude from Yale and then Harvard Medical School and planned to become a general practitioner just like his father. But then, continuing his medical training at Massachusetts General Hospital, he assisted the famous paediatric surgeon W. Hardy Hendren on an operation. A child had been born with congenital diaphragmatic hernia, a defect in which the baby's diaphragm – the sheet of muscle separating the chest and the abdomen – develops with a hole, which allows the abdominal organs to rise into the chest, stopping the lungs developing. Hendren's surgery to repair the hernia was immaculate, yet the child died. The cause of death was blindingly obvious to Harrison. It wasn't the anatomical problem of the hole in the diaphragm per se – it was the way this defect had compressed the lungs in utero, not giving them a chance to grow. 'The only way to save that kid was to fix the problem before birth,' Harrison told Hendren. Hendren was so shocked by Harrison's ludicrous naivety, he almost fell down.[3] But a touch of ludicrous naivety can be the mark of a genius.

Harrison thought about his idea for a number of years. Finally, in the new year of 1978, he got his chance. He took up a faculty position at the University of California at San Francisco, an unstuffy and open-minded institution[4] where researchers were unhampered by too much regulatory red tape.[5] Here he at last had the resources and freedom to explore his question: could babies with congenital defects be operated on before birth – before it was too late?

In fact the idea of open surgery on unborn babies – cutting open the womb, operating on the fetus, then resealing the womb – wasn't totally new. Animal fetuses were used as experimental models in the 1960s and 1970s and there had, in the early 1960s, been a few first attempts at open fetal surgery on humans in New York and Puerto Rico.[6] These ill-fated transfusion procedures involved a risky abdominal operation on the mother to expose the uterus and give the baby a blood transfusion before closing the womb again. In a pre-ultrasound era, with no way for the surgeon to see the fetus clearly, the results were dire, and nobody had attempted it since.[7]

But Harrison – frustrated as a baby doctor by 'seeing problems in newborn babies that were too late to fix'[8] – believed it could be done. Michael Harrison remains a rather mysterious figure to me. I requested an interview with him for this book several times but received no reply. I was advised by those who know him that I would never get any response, that Dr Harrison, now a grandfather in his mid-seventies, had not only retired from the field (to research the use of magnets in surgery instead) but also was not remotely interested in talking to journalists.[9] I already knew this, having read his extraordinary textbooks. From the start, Harrison barred the press from his operating rooms and laboratories, aware that his work could easily be (and was) sensationalized. He wanted to focus on the needs of families, not perform ' "spectacular" fetal interventions for media attention.'[10]

Harrison was a fun maverick, by all accounts. When another guru of fetal medicine, the British Greek-Cypriot Kypros Nicolaides, told me about his last meeting with Michael Harrison, at a hamburger joint in California when Harrison was around seventy, his face softened. 'When I saw him I felt sad. When I looked at him walk into the room, this full-of-energy guy, now, he's walking slowly. And then he sat down, and the guy started speaking.' Nicolaides snapped his fingers. 'I said to myself: "this guy is twenty-two".'

'In his mind?' I asked. 'Yes!' grinned Nicolaides. 'This guy is completely mad. He's brilliant.'

Harrison started a team, including a protégé, Scott Adzick – a trainee paediatric surgeon ten years his junior, who joined him as a research fellow – as well as a bright young children's nurse called Lori Howell. Together they were determined to convince the world – and themselves – that fetal surgery could save babies. When Harrison and Adzick presented the idea at medical conferences, they were virtually laughed out of the room. 'There was a huge amount of scepticism – huge,' Adzick later remembered. 'We walked off the stage thinking maybe we are crazy . . . but –' he narrowed his blue eyes, deadly serious – 'we weren't.'[11]

They experimented on thousands of pregnant sheep and monkeys, making things up as they went.[12] No idea was off limits.[13] One major problem they had to solve was how to open and close the pregnant uterus. You might imagine opening the womb to be as straightforward as a C-section, but in the middle of pregnancy (as opposed to full term) the uterus is thick and packed with blood vessels. As for closing it, it was like closing a water balloon without a leak.[14] Conventional surgical staples, they found, acted like an IUD, a coil which prevents pregnancy – so a stapling device had to be developed which quickly cut through the wall of the uterus, firing off absorbable staples to pinch off its large blood vessels.[15]

The failures outnumbered the successes. But finally, cautiously, in isolated cases where there was no other hope for the baby, they started to work with human fetuses – being honest with the families about what they could and could not do, what their hopes were, and what their fears were. The first child to undergo totally experimental fetal surgery in 1981 had an obstruction in the urinary tract. It sounds a small defect, but in a fetus this destroys the developing kidneys so that once born they could spend years on a kidney machine – the lungs could also be damaged, and babies could die.[16] Unblocking a *born* baby's bladder would be a pretty straightforward operation – so could it not be done in utero, and save a life that would otherwise end before it began?

In this first operation, Harrison managed to make a new hole in the urinary tract to circumvent the blockage, but sadly, by the time the operation came, it was too late for the child. The kidneys had failed already and the lungs had been stunted by a lack of amniotic fluid. Death followed soon after birth.[17]

Then Rosa Skinner came along – forty-two years old and pregnant with twins. The girl twin was healthy, but the boy was found to have a blockage in his urethra, preventing him from passing urine. By the time Rosa was seven months pregnant, her son's belly was blown up like a football; his lungs and kidneys were at severe risk. The stakes for Harrison this time were even higher: under ultrasound guidance, he had to pull an unborn boy's bottom half out of a pregnant woman's uterus and insert a shunt into its bladder to redirect urine out into the amniotic cavity, without harming his twin.[18] 'We were just in agony,' Harrison later recalled of this ethical dilemma. As for Rosa, she was to recall, 'All I knew was that my babies were in trouble . . . I put it in God's hands.'

It was the first successful open operation on a human fetus and the twins were born two weeks later, on Mother's Day 1981 – Mary, and Michael, named after the surgeon.[19] Michael Skinner urinated through the new hole the surgeons had created until he was six months old, and then his bladder was repaired. He grew up healthy.[20]

Only 41 per cent of fetuses with blocked bladders survived after a fetal shunt in the early days of the 1980s,[21] but even a low success rate meant a lot of saved lives. Harrison realized shunts could help other conditions, too. He soon tried shunts in babies with hydrocephalus (water on the brain) and hydrops. The former was a disaster[22] – although most of the fetuses who had fetal brain surgery survived, more than half were left with severe neurological disability.[23] But the latter idea ultimately led to the sort of shunt which saved my own son's life.

In his *Atlas of Fetal Surgery* – a book he wrote in 1996 detailing the experiments he did that got this field off the ground – Harrison comes across as a one-of-a-kind character. The book is full of images: an illustration of a grinning fetal monkey in a bikini; a diagram showing a sleeping anaesthetized mother monkey, her uterus opened with a stapler and her baby's bottom half pulled out for surgery. One photograph shows a scrawny little monkey who has undergone a fetal procedure: arms and legs flailing, neck encircled by a human hand, his eyes blindfolded. In a caption, Harrison wrote that the monkey 'prefers to remain anonymous'.[24]

Harrison clearly cared profoundly for the people he treated. Calling the fetus 'our most reticent patient', he wrote: 'Only now are we beginning to consider the fetus seriously – medically, legally, and ethically . . . The short but eventful history of the fetus as a patient reassures us that fetal treatment offers new hope for the fetus with a correctable defect, and reminds us that there is considerable potential for doing harm.'[25] As for the other patient – the pregnant mother or the 'innocent bystander' as Harrison called her – he saw her safety as paramount.[26] 'A fetal abnormality of any type should never be treated simply "because it is there", and never by someone who is unprepared for this fearsome responsibility,' Harrison reflected in 2001. 'In the early harrowing days of fetal treatment, no one could be sure whether the enterprise would succeed or die.'[27]

Dr N. Scott Adzick (his official name: the N stands for Nick – but his colleagues and friends call him Scott) and Lori Howell eventually set up their own Center for Fetal Diagnosis and Treatment at CHOP in 1995, where they have continued to come up with creative solutions to seemingly insoluble problems.[28] CHOP – the first children's hospital in America, founded in 1855 – is the American equivalent of Britain's Great Ormond Street Hospital (GOSH) and has a similar position in the university district of a big grey city, but it's a confident, punchy place that makes GOSH look laid back. To get an appointment you dial 800-IN-UTERO. In an all-American way, the staff are justifiably proud of their unit's reputation as the world leader in fetal surgery under Adzick.

The fetal medicine patients here don't have to labour alongside ordinary mothers. They have fetal surgery in an operating room, give birth in their own special delivery unit, and if their baby needs an operation or neonatal care after birth, that's also done on site. There are no junior doctors in this fetal unit, only consultants. The nurses in the neonatal unit wear smart grey uniforms, the doctors wear white coats with their names embroidered on in cursive script, and everyone is well groomed.

Patients have been coming here from all over America (and places like Dubai) for nearly a quarter of a century now. If parents can't cover the costs with their insurance, CHOP will try to find a way to fund their treatment. Many patients arrive here with an incorrect diagnosis from their local hospital.

Some have been advised to terminate when there is still a good chance for their baby – here, they may be given an option they didn't have before, to have a procedure or even an operation before birth.

*

The British have always regarded the open fetal surgery practised in America with some wariness. British doctors have linked the millions of dollars of funding Harrison raised for his animal experiments to anti-abortion lobbyists, who hoped that fixing congenital disorders in utero would mean fewer terminations.[29]

Beyond this, some of the early open fetal surgery experiments around the world were disasters, too frequently ending in deaths, the British thought. The pioneering British fetal medics were obstetricians; the Americans were paediatric surgeons. The British, ultimately preferring to work with minimally invasive techniques performed with needles – like my shunt – felt that the Americans, being surgeons, were somewhat knife-happy.[30] I'm not sure if this is fair, though: the Americans were all too aware of the massive dangers of open fetal surgery. Harrison and Adzick have always preferred minimally invasive surgical techniques[31] and of course, first invented many of them (including Joel's shunt).

Most of the work at CHOP is minimally invasive. And sometimes, knowledge means deciding not to intervene. Lori Howell, the warm and motherly children's nurse with long brown hair who was part of Harrison and Adzick's core team from the early days and is now executive director of the Center for Fetal Diagnosis and Treatment at CHOP, told me about 'gut-wrenching counselling sessions where parents literally beg you for the procedure and we've known it's not the right thing to do'.

Controversy over both the safety and politics of open fetal surgery is still raging across the world, and the clinical ethics of fetal medicine are still in their infancy – for example, as I'll come to later, giving a fetus anaesthesia is not a given, even today – but there are one or two types of open fetal surgery which are now gaining international, mainstream acceptance.

One, the EXIT (ex utero intrapartum treatment) procedure, could be described as a C-section to the next level. The operation was developed by Michael Harrison as a response to what he called the 'dark side'[32] of attempts to repair one of the most dangerous fetal illnesses, congenital diaphragmatic hernia (CDH).

No one knows yet why CDH happens, but it occurs in about one in 2,500 babies, at around the third month of pregnancy.[33] The lungs develop abnormally, partly because they are squashed by the abdominal organs migrating into the chest, and at birth the baby is unable to breathe. Only a century ago a medical textbook described the condition as 'usually found in monsters'.[34]

Harrison and Adzick originally experimented with repairing CDH in the womb as a surgeon would after birth – opening the womb, cutting into the baby, rearranging the chest organs, stitching up the diaphragm and putting the baby back in the womb.

Ever since he first had the idea of repairing defects in utero in the 1970s, CDH had been the one thing Michael Harrison wanted to fix.[35] But the problem seemed frustratingly unfixable.[36] In the most serious cases of CDH, the liver moves up into the chest. The fetal surgeons discovered there was an insurmountable technical obstacle in trying to move it back in utero. When they pushed the liver back down out of the chest during open fetal surgery, the umbilical vein (the fetal lifeline which delivers oxygenated blood from the mother's placenta to the baby's heart), which passes through the liver, became kinked and could not recover. As they moved the liver, the surgeons would hear the terrible, telltale slowing of the fetal pulse on the monitor, like a battery winding down: 'beepbeepbeep . . . beep . . . beep . . . buuup . . . buuup . . . . . . buuuup . . . . . .'[37] Babies died.

Finally forced to give up on his efforts with this method, Harrison came up with a 'counter-intuitive' idea in the 1990s. It was, perhaps, his cleverest idea of all, and has gradually spread around the world. Back in the mid-1980s, he and Adzick had found a way to make fetal lungs grow in animal experiments – by blocking the tube between the throat and the windpipe and lungs – the trachea – with a clip. This sounds inimical to saving a life, but the baby doesn't need its airways to breathe until birth. Instead the fetal lung makes fluid, which normally streams out through the trachea into the amniotic sac or is swallowed. This tracheal fluid maintains an important pressure which keeps the lungs developing. If there is not enough fluid, the pressure in the airways goes down and the lungs fail to grow. But if you temporarily block the trachea in utero, animal studies showed, the lungs continue to make fluid, the pressure goes up, and this induces lung growth. Now, Harrison and Adzick realized they could use this airway blocking procedure to save fetuses with CDH. These babies' lungs were producing fluid normally, but the lungs were small and underdeveloped, partly because they were squashed by the organs moving into the chest. The idea was to place a clip on the trachea during open fetal surgery so the lungs would grow, and then to remove the clip in a second operation before birth.

The organs in the chest would be rearranged in another operation after birth.

Today, the procedure in utero is done as keyhole surgery,[†]
with the mother awake and watching the camera's eye-view
on a big screen. The surgeon inserts a hollow cannula through
the mother's abdomen into her uterus. They then feed a tiny
camera through the baby's mouth and blow up a minuscule
balloon – the kind used to block off burst blood vessels in
brain surgery – into the child's trachea, just below the vocal
cords, to plug the airways. The plug prevents tracheal fluid
from leaking out, which in turn makes the lungs expand and
allows the lungs to inflate and grow.[38] Then, in a second procedure, the balloon is removed just before a planned birth, so
the baby can breathe when born.

What is this like for the mother? Sophie, a recent British
patient, a quiet, sensible woman in her thirties with wavy
brown hair, is a senior hospital doctor herself, in a field unre-
lated to obstetrics. She told me that even for her as a doctor,
'It's absolutely the stuff of science fiction.' In Sophie's words:
'I'm an insider in the medical field, but what they do in the
fetal medicine unit is something I'd never seen. I didn't know
they could get away with it.'

The point at which Sophie's pregnancy went haywire came
twenty-five weeks in. She and her husband Chris already had
a healthy toddler, Andrew. At a scan at their local hospital, the
sonographer had a feeling that something wasn't right with the
baby's heart, even though it looked structurally normal. He
sent Sophie for a scan of the baby's heart at their nearest fetal
medicine unit. There the cardiologist immediately realized

†   This operation was pioneered by Professor Jan Deprest, another
leading fetal surgeon, based at Leuven University in Belgium.

what was wrong. The heart was normal but had been pushed into the left-hand side of the chest by CDH.

Because she is a doctor, Sophie immediately knew how serious this was. Chris, who works in property, stood next to her saying, 'Aren't you glad everything's all right with the heart?' But Sophie burst into tears. The chance of dying at birth for a baby with CDH is usually around 50–50,[39] but it was worse in Sophie and Chris's case because right-sided CDH is rarer and more severe. Their baby's chance of living was more like one in five, they were told.

The day of the diagnosis, they were immediately offered a termination, but this religious couple would not consider that. So they agreed to the procedure. Medical staff come from all over the world to watch such things, and Sophie was asked for consent for what turned out to be around twelve observers in the operating room. Sophie and Chris were told to ignore all the people watching and only interact with the brisk consultant in fetal medicine who would carry out the intervention, and his registrar.

Terrified and shaking, Sophie said to the doctor, 'What if I move?'

He said, 'I don't care if you move.'

The operation started with an amniocentesis and, under ultrasound, the consultant stabbed general anaesthetic into the baby's thigh to ensure total stillness. Sophie felt 'a really weird thing – pain in my stomach when he stabbed the baby with the anaesthetic needle. I shouldn't have felt anything. I think I was tensing up because I could see what he was doing on the ultrasound.' The room waited for the baby to fall asleep – he kept turning and turning. The atmosphere was kept upbeat, the doctor joking, 'Is the baby asleep yet?' and tapping Sophie's stomach to see if the baby responded. Finally, he stopped moving.

The consultant made another cut and fed the fetoscope into the uterus, then threaded the camera in through it. He had to find the baby's mouth. Seeing her child's face from the camera's viewpoint was amazing to Sophie. The camera went into the mouth and then the surgeon pushed in the balloon and inflated it with water. It was painful for Sophie; her uterus started contracting.

Yet she was silent – 'so terrified of moving and making him lose his position'. She told me: 'I cried right the way through, silently, tears rolling down my face; my husband there with a tissue, mopping each side.'

As you'd expect, there were serious risks of infection and setting off labour. Sophie stopped work afterwards and had to wear a medical alert bracelet at all times to warn that her baby had a balloon in his airways, in case she collapsed and her baby was born unexpectedly.

For three weeks, Sophie had weekly scans and her baby's lungs seemed to be getting bigger, although the outcome was still very uncertain. Then, suddenly, at twenty-nine weeks' gestation, her waters broke.

'We had some horrible discussions,' Sophie told me. 'The neonatal team said, "Well, what do you want us to do?", as in "Would you want us to leave him, or do you want us to stick him with needles and try and resuscitate?" We were all for resuscitation, even though they were saying there was basically no chance. We needed to know that we'd tried everything.' The doctors told her and Chris that they would try, but they warned the couple that the baby might not make it off the resuscitation table.

The surgeon took out the balloon, so that when the baby

came, the neonatologists could try resuscitation. That Christmas, while her son Andrew had his second birthday, Sophie stayed in hospital, amniotic fluid leaking out of her but not in labour, for ten more days. No one knew what to do with her, and she felt miserable. At home, her parents moved in to look after Andrew so Chris could spend time at the hospital.

The consultant decided to try to put the balloon in a second time, something he had never tried to do before except in cases where the first balloon had burst. It was pretty uncharted territory and would bring further risks, but could also give the baby's lungs better growth. This time, even more people were watching the procedure. Sophie was 'terrified by the advancement of everything' – she 'wanted to freeze time'. It was hard to believe, in a way, that her baby really was critically ill, when she had been hugging her belly and feeling him kicking. The baby seemed, to her, safe inside. If only time would stop. As Sophie told me this, she silently shed a few tears.

She said to one of the consultants: 'It goes against every instinct in my maternal body to let you come at my stomach with an enormous 25 centimetre-long needle.' Everything a mother does in pregnancy is to keep that baby safe. In undergoing fetal surgeries, Sophie found, 'there was such a lot to suppress'.

At thirty-three weeks, another scan found Sophie's cervix was shortening, a sign labour could be imminent. The doctors took the balloon out a second time, so the baby would be able to breathe on delivery. But the procedure pushed Sophie firmly into labour. She had been desperate for the baby not to be born premature, but he was coming.

As Sophie's story shows, lifesaving fetal procedures place mothers at high risk of another serious danger: premature labour. If a fetus with a blockage in the airways is born unexpectedly, it will of course be unable to breathe – it would be impossible to operate to unblock the airways fast enough. But Harrison had a solution for this too. What if you could buy time to unblock the baby's trachea *during birth itself,* by operating while the baby was still attached to the placenta and kept alive by it? So in the early 1990s, looking for a way to save babies with a CDH clip and thus at high risk of being born prematurely, before the second operation to unblock the airways, Harrison developed the operation called EXIT – ever-whimsical, he also called it 'OOPS', short for operating on placental support.[40]

If a mother went into premature labour, the uterus could be opened under general anaesthetic and the baby partially delivered, as if by C-section – but the baby would be left attached to the placenta through the umbilical cord while surgeons removed the plug and ensured there was an airway for the child to breathe through. Only then would the umbilical cord be severed and the child delivered.

Today, the fetoscopic balloon treatment for CDH has reduced the risk of premature labour enough that the EXIT procedure need only be used rarely in CDH cases, in an emergency when the balloon cannot be removed using other techniques. But this has by no means been the end of EXIT. It has become an increasingly popular planned operation in other dire situations – after Scott Adzick realized that the same technique could be used for babies who have blocked airways for different reasons. One of these is called CHAOS.

CHAOS stands for congenital higher airway obstruction syndrome, a rare fetal condition. A congenital blockage in the unborn baby's airway means it can't breathe and swallow amniotic fluid properly. The overflowing airways swell the lungs, and the heart is squashed by amniotic fluid, leading to hydrops and death.

This is not the sort of problem you read about in pregnancy manuals; not the kind of problem any expectant parent imagines. One couple as unsuspecting as any others were Jess and Will: busy, active thirty-something Londoners who both worked in business. Until twenty-six weeks into Jess's first pregnancy, life was normal, but she was to become an EXIT patient, and to find that despite expert care and planning, things can get scarier than even the doctors imagine too.

When a midwife thought Jess was measuring bigger than expected, she referred Jess to her local hospital for a scan. The baby appeared to have hydrops and his lungs looked unusual. Finally, Jess and Will were sent to the fetal medicine unit at UCH, and a diagnosis of CHAOS was given with 90 per cent probability.

EXIT, a rare and risky operation on a fetus during delivery, could possibly save this baby. At the time of writing, only seven EXIT procedures have been done at UCH, and five of these babies survived. Mr Pandya explained to Jess and Will how once the baby reached thirty-four weeks, they could deliver the baby's head and shoulders, and perform a temporary tracheostomy – make a hole in the throat – while the baby was also still getting oxygen from the placenta. Once the baby could breathe air, they would deliver the rest of his body. All this would take place under a general anaesthetic for Jess and the baby. Later, the doctors could find the exact obstruction in the baby's airways and operate to fix it. Such an obscure problem is still not possible to detect through scans of a tiny baby in utero.

There were a couple of other options. Jess could deliver her baby naturally, vaginally, and doctors could try to unblock the airways at birth, but, unable to take a breath of air, the child was likely to die before they could do so. The only other option was to terminate. By this time, Jess was twenty-eight weeks pregnant. An injection would be given to stop the baby's heartbeat and she would have to deliver him.

Waiting for the EXIT procedure sounds like the obvious decision, but it wasn't that simple. Because the EXIT procedure can only be done once the baby reaches thirty-four weeks, the baby's critical condition in the weeks before then could lead to premature labour (and death), or heart failure (and death). Also, there was no certainty about the child's life even if it was saved. Would he be able to breathe in the end, to eat and drink, to speak?

An EXIT procedure is a big deal to set up. Multiple consultants – 'the A team', as Pandya put it – need to clear their diaries. Twenty to thirty doctors would be working in the A team, including fetal doctors, neonatologists and anaesthetists for both mother and baby. 'Because it was so highly medicalized, sometimes the pregnancy didn't seem all ours,' Jess told me.

The day finally came, at thirty-five weeks. Jess and Will took the underground into UCH at the break of day. As Jess sat in her hospital gown, many of the doctors came to say hello. Everyone seemed to know Jess. One doctor said: 'You're going to meet your baby today.' She walked into the operating theatre in the labour ward, lay down on the tilting bed usually used for caesareans, and felt suddenly intimidated.

Will watched as his wife was anaesthetized deeply enough to anaesthetize the baby too. It was a horrible thing to witness. In a way, it was harder for Will than for Jess, because there wasn't a lot he could do, and he had to be the strong one. He started to cry, and a midwife led him outside.

When Jess woke, groggy, a sweet-faced neonatologist called Giles Kendall was by her side. Jess pointed at her throat to ask if they had done the tracheostomy on the baby. Dr Kendall gently said no, they hadn't been able to do that.

The EXIT itself had gone smoothly. They couldn't find a blockage in the airways. The baby was delivered. It had all gone well enough at first.

But the baby's lungs wouldn't fill with air. The doctors were mystified. Why couldn't they keep him oxygenated? The little boy's blood oxygen levels were at just 30 per cent and he was brain damaged already.

He wasn't going to make it. They had woken Jess up so she could hold him.

She was wheeled in her bed into another room where she waited a little while with Will. They named their son Corey. Telling me about this, Jess's memory blurred. She remembered being placed next to Corey who was being scanned, attached to various machines. Then the doctors told the parents there was nothing more they could do. They unplugged him from the machines, and passed him in a blanket to Jess, and then Will. Giles Kendall placed his stethoscope over Corey's chest. He had gone.

On the day of Corey's death, Jess couldn't cry, couldn't respond emotionally to what was happening. She stayed in hospital for three days, not leaving her room in the labour ward. 'It was such a weird place to be, there with Corey, feeling locked in this room and not knowing what to do. I didn't think about what was outside the door.'

A post-mortem eventually found that Corey's lungs had never formed properly. They were solid, so they didn't take in air and expand like a balloon. And there was only one pulmonary vein, when there should have been four. It was a vanishingly rare, random malformation.

The fact that their baby died didn't in any way lessen this family's respect for the doctors who were unable to save him. If anything, a bond grew up between them after the tragedy. The doctors truly cared, and still do today.

'Even though I look after lots of babies who do die at some stage,' Mr Pandya told me when we discussed Corey's case, 'I don't often see the actual death.' After Corey died, Mr Pandya called Jess and Will at home. 'You're still in my thoughts,' he told them. Two years later, he showed me a card he still treasures in his desk, which Jess wrote thanking him and his team for all they did to save Corey. The family still visits him at least once a year at the unit.

Jess – usually sociable – kept away from friends and family for a while after this loss. 'They were happy, they had children, and we didn't. People didn't know what to say to us. Some people didn't even mention Corey to us.'

But after Corey died, some of the doctors, in shock themselves at what had happened, came to see Jess once or twice a day in hospital. It seemed to Jess that the medics were the one group of people who really understood what she was going through.

*

EXIT is a halfway-house kind of open fetal surgery – it's audacious, but at the end, the baby is not sealed back into the womb, but delivered. The other experiment in open fetal surgery which is now spreading around the world is perhaps even bolder and more alien.

This operation was first done successfully in 1997, at CHOP, and I flew there in the summer of 2018 to witness it myself.

On the morning of the operation I was allowed to observe, I arrived at 7.15 a.m., having hardly slept and feeling anxious. I hadn't yet met Dr Adzick apart from a quick hello, and now I was to watch him in theatre. As I gowned up to step into the fetal operating theatre, my mask had to be tied just so. There was no pool of mismatched plastic Crocs for scrubs here as I had once noticed at Great Ormond Street Hospital – the staff in CHOP's operating theatre wore their own shiny black shoes. I stood as unobtrusively as I could in a corner of the theatre, taking in around twenty doctors and nurses milling around the patients: a mother in her early thirties and the twenty-five-week-old baby she was carrying. My view of the mother was obscured by the crowd of surgeons around her but I could just see her belly swabbed with brown disinfectant and her arm taped down, her fingers slightly curled. Her face was hidden behind blue drapes. A warm bath of saline solution stood beside her feet. She had already been given a deep anaesthetic, deep enough to relax the uterus completely and anaesthetize the baby.

Despite so many staff – including fetal surgeons, obstetricians, anaesthetists and a fetal cardiologist who would monitor the baby's heart continually – the room was silent.

The surgeons – Scott Adzick, Alan Flake and Holly Hedrick – opened the mother's abdomen with a Bovie, an electric cauterizing device that blows cells apart to cut tissue and simultaneously dehydrates the cells, which stops the cut tissue bleeding. A smell of burning flesh seeped into the air. With giant retractors, the mother's abdomen was opened and the uterus popped up like popcorn, pink and round. The next step was to locate the placenta using an ultrasound probe – the surgeons needed to avoid touching and damaging it at all costs. Then, with the Bovie, they opened the uterus. Amniotic fluid bubbled then poured out, but the doctors infused fluid at body temperature back in to replace it and keep the fetus warm and buoyant.

Now, they cut a diamond shape in the uterus with the special stapling device Adzick had helped invent, and immediately the baby's back came into view on the monitor I was watching – a wall of pink flesh.

This tiny unborn person, the size of a mug of coffee, had been diagnosed with a condition many parents around the world fear, and some terminate for. Spina bifida is less common in developed countries than it used to be now pregnant women know to take folic acid, which helps prevent it, but it still happens. Early in pregnancy, the fetus develops a neural tube – a structure which later becomes the brain and spinal cord, crucial to the body's nervous system. Normally, the tube closes four weeks after conception, but in spina bifida, part of the tube fails to close. In the most severe cases – the kind they do fetal surgery for – the baby's spinal cord ends up pushed out of its back in a little sac. The damage caused by spina bifida in the womb can lead to leg paralysis, incontinence and lack of sensation in the lower half of the body, as well as brain damage.[41]

Normally, a neurosurgeon operates to close the neural tube defect after the baby is born, but in the mid-1990s, fetal medics came up with the idea that the open neural tube could be closed off in utero, before too much damage was done. The operation has to be done before twenty-six weeks, because later in pregnancy, the baby's urine takes on a different chemical composition which, when spina bifida is untreated, starts to attack the exposed spinal cord and nerve tissue. It's at this stage that irreparable damage occurs. Spina bifida surgery in

utero dramatically changed the outlook for babies. If babies
are operated on prenatally for spina bifida they are twice as
likely to be able to walk as the children operated on post-
natally. Prenatal surgery also lessens the risk of spina bifida
causing brain damage.[42] At CHOP, families are given all
three options: to have the fetal surgery, to have postnatal surgery, or to terminate – and some do still terminate. There is
no judgement, whatever they do. 'No matter which one
they're going to choose, they're going to do it because they
love their baby,' the warm and down-to-earth fetal neurosurgeon Greg Heuer told me.

He knows what families go through. He and his wife were
once fetal medicine patients themselves and lost one of their
twins. Greg, a proud family man who has photos of his daughter displayed in his office, told me he treats the babies he
operates on as if they are his own children. He vividly recalls
the first time he operated on a fetus and thought: 'We shouldn't
be able to do that.' Fetal surgery still seems weird to him. He
said to me, 'The idea is crazy. It doesn't make any sense that
this could work. Dr Adzick was told for years that he was
insane.' Fetal surgery, he added, 'is like buying Christmas presents in February. You have to be very organized, and you
don't see the reward for months.'

The surgeons pushed a tube into the fetus to give it an extra
shot of anaesthetic, and they infused fluid into the amniotic
sac to fool the mother's body into assuming the pregnancy was
not compromised. The dark line of the child's spinal cord was
visible, an open gash shaped like a horseshoe exposing a knob
of tissue where the spina bifida sac had ended up ballooning
out of the baby's skin. Now, with another surgeon holding the
baby's back in place, and second-by-second monitoring of the
baby's vital signs, Greg Heuer took over, incising the sac next

to the spinal cord, releasing the pressure of cerebrospinal fluid which had stretched the cord and sac through the skin. Without the pressure, the spinal cord slipped naturally back into the spinal canal where it was supposed to be. Heuer then had to mend the exposure just as he would if operating after birth, but making allowances for the far more fragile flesh of the unborn, which is not much better at holding a stitch than wet tissue paper.[43]

Heuer had to close the flesh in layers – first the meninges, the membranes around the spinal cord; then the muscles and connective tissue; then the skin. I watched him using tweezers and scissors to pull gently at the flesh on either side of the opening to draw out flaps of tissue. Then, like lacing shoes or a corset, he drew the flaps neatly together with a few sutures, closing the neural tube away where it should be, beneath the skin. It was, essentially, needlework.

They try to keep operations on fetuses under ninety minutes at CHOP because this reduces the chance of preterm labour.[44] Thirty-seven minutes into this surgery and the baby's back was stitched up. It had been a straightforward success thanks to the well-oiled team; they had made it look bizarrely easy. I sensed an instant relief in the room the second the fetus was no longer open, like a letting out of breath. People started to murmur a little louder and walked less stiffly. They started to tail off the mother's anaesthesia – she would be woken as soon as her abdomen was closed. She wouldn't need painkillers after a day or two.

Half the medical team now disappeared. All that remained now was to sew the uterus back together and push it back in, covering it with a layer of yellow fat. The entire operation, like a puzzle of Russian dolls, had taken just over an hour. In four days, if all continued well, the mother would be discharged, to spend the rest of her pregnancy on bed rest, before a very care-ful C-section just before term, to avoid the risk of natural labour for a mother whose womb has already been cut open. 'Now the real work starts – she has to keep the baby in,' Lori Howell told me, putting her hand on my shoulder. This after-math is the toughest part, in a way, of fetal surgery. Violating the membranes around the baby presents a serious risk. Very, very rarely, a surgery goes smoothly, but the next day, the baby's heartbeat can't be found, and the child is stillborn. Others have been born so prematurely they cannot survive.[45]

As the 2010s come to a close, open fetal surgery for spina bifida is gradually spreading around the world. Only around thirty fetal medicine units globally offer it at the time of writing, almost all clustered in the USA and Western Europe – though there are a few outposts in Peru, Australia and Iran. Apart from at the most established open fetal surgery centres – for example in Philadelphia, San Francisco, Belgium, Switzerland and Poland – at many others (like UCH, which in 2018, in partnership with Great Ormond Street Hospital, per-formed the first open fetal surgeries for spina bifida in Britain) the number of times this surgery has been performed are at the time of writing countable on one or two hands.[46] It's a fast-moving field – as the NHS starts rolling out this open fetal surgery for spina bifida, in some hospitals, it's already being replaced by a less invasive procedure.[47]

A few hours after the operation I watched – which I later learned resulted in the birth at thirty-seven weeks of a healthy baby who required no further operations and had good leg movements – I waited outside Scott Adzick's office for a twenty-five-minute slot with him, clutching a humble gift of a tin of biscuits, shaking like a schoolchild about to see the headmaster. Greg Heuer had joked to me: 'He knows my wife's birthday. He knows everything . . . he will know more about you than you know about you.' My heart was racing.

Adzick appeared, a tall, bluff Midwesterner with silver hair and white teeth. His office was decorated with baseball photos and on a wooden table lay a gift from a patient, a framed maxim by Calvin Coolidge to put on the wall which read: 'Nothing in the world can take the place of persistence'. Dr Adzick gets up at 5 a.m. and is at the hospital by 6.30 a.m. each day, works till late, and likes to stay fit.

His original motivation to become a surgeon was his own mother, who was diagnosed with breast cancer when he was a boy of eleven. After a radical mastectomy and radiation therapy, she survived, and her son was so grateful to her surgeon that he decided to be a surgeon when he grew up.[48]

I asked Dr Adzick to describe himself to me. He replied: 'Dr Relentless.'

'That's a bit of an understatement,' laughed Ashley, the hospital PR, sitting by my side.

When I met Dr Adzick, his own granddaughter Annie had just been born at his special delivery unit – she had been growing small, and, not getting the answers he wanted at the hospital where she was being monitored, he had her transferred here, where he oversaw her safety and she made a 'spectacular debut'. 'Can you imagine having him as your grandfather?' smiled Ashley.

When I asked Dr Adzick if he could tell me about cases he had worked on in the early days, he murmured in his fast, unostentatious voice, 'If you're looking for drama, I'm not gonna give it to you.'

'I understand,' I said. 'I don't want to sensationalize either.' I tried to explain this book was serious, but I was faced with silence. I could see why Dr Adzick might still feel wary of me as a journalist, despite having so generously welcomed me to observe him in the operating theatre, a privilege I was told few are granted. He is a hero to many, and his staff and patients treat him like a king, yet he has also spent much of his professional career being told he is a crazy risk-taker.

The more I spoke to Dr Adzick about medical facts, the more he relaxed. He wished me luck with my book, and I noticed he had a slight stammer which made him seem suddenly less intimidating. Towards the end of our time together, Dr Adzick's eyes lit up. He was telling me how much it means to him to see the children he has operated on grow up. We spoke about Maeve, whom he operated on for SCT. 'That kid is just totally awesome,' Adzick said, no longer swallowing his words, the timbre of his voice lifting. 'You look at that kid and you have to marvel.'

He continued: 'It's not what our team did or what I did . . . certain things you just can't explain.' Children like Maeve, he said, 'maybe they're just lucky, maybe they're just incredibly resilient. But I believe in miracles.'

Then, thinking more, he added firmly, 'There's no magic formula. I don't think it's luck. It's preparation. It's some good fortune. It's resilience. It's relentlessness. It is not giving in, not giving up. It's going from failure to failure with undiminished enthusiasm.'

3

Stabs in the Dark

'The fetus could not be taken seriously as long as he remained a medical recluse in an opaque womb; and it was not until the last half of this century that the prying eye of the ultrasonogram rendered the once opaque womb transparent, stripping the veil of mystery from the dark inner sanctum, and letting the light of scientific observation fall on the shy and secretive fetus.'

MICHAEL HARRISON, THE 'FATHER' OF FETAL SURGERY, 2001[1]

There's not much to see in the fetal medicine unit – to the naked eye, at least. Just a waiting room and some scanning suites. All the drama, all the action, is hidden behind those suites' closed doors – and then beyond that, hidden in the amniotic sac of each pregnant woman, unseeable to anyone except the doctors with their black and white scanning machines broadcasting fuzzy pictures. One bump looks much like another, but the scans reveal that every bump has its story. The baby's underwater heartbeat, measured with the Doppler scanner, sounds with an unearthly 'wow wow', like a signal from the depths of the ocean or space. So close, and yet so far away. The heart's rhythm makes patterns on the screen – arcs, waves, electrical flashes of red and blue. The doctors' expressions, dictated by these flashes and arcs, are blasé, or intent with concern.

To understand how fetal surgery even became a possibility, you have to stretch further back in time. Until extremely recently, the fetus was an unreachable mystery, a secret locked inside a woman's body. The earliest known illustrations of a fetus in utero, dating back to the thirteenth century, show tiny, fully formed people doing gymnastics inside a jar.[2] For hundreds of years it was believed that these miniature preformed human beings – homunculi, Latin for 'little men' – were contained within each sperm or egg, and simply grew in size.[3]

And for centuries, the only reliable knowledge of the unborn came from autopsies of miscarried or aborted babies, or from animal experiments.[4] At the turn of the nineteenth century, the commonest way of referring to an expected baby was as a 'little stranger'.[5] As for a baby born with an abnormality, theories in centuries past ranged from the mother creating deformities with her troubled thoughts to heaven-sent warnings. *Tractatus de Monstris* – Latin for *Treatise about Monsters* – a 1570 book by French bishop Arnaud Sorbin, was filled with woodcut illustrations of babies said to have been born with extreme (and unlikely) malformations, including extra pairs of eyes and ears, or four feet. The bishop saw these 'monsters' as portents from heaven; caused by human sin.[6] In the eighteenth century, wax and clay models of babies with abnormalities were made for a new school of obstetrics in Bologna, Italy, where they were used as teaching examples of 'monstrous birth'. The school's founder, obstetrician Giovanni Galli, lectured on the power of the maternal imagination to deform the fetus.[7] It was not until very recently that attitudes to disability changed. Even in 1931, a Great Ormond Street Hospital paediatrician, writing about Sorbin and his monsters, commented, 'those may be right who regarded these strange monsters as somehow connected with the antichrist'.[8]

The only way to get to the human fetus is through the mother. Sticking a sharp needle into a woman's abdomen with a baby inside, but without any way of knowing where it will end up, seems insane today, but this was done until the early 1970s. The earliest gynaecological operations in America were for ectopic pregnancies, where a baby grows in the fallopian tubes, a dangerous condition which, if left untreated, can kill the mother when the amniotic sac runs out of space to expand and ruptures. The only treatment is to abort the pregnancy, and cutting a fetus out was done successfully – the mother surviving – as early as 1759.[9] It seems the first surgical attempt to treat, rather than abort, a fetus in the womb was 'amnio-drainage' – draining the womb of excess amniotic fluid after puncturing it with a needle – first performed in the 1880s in cases of polyhydramnios, where there is too much amniotic fluid and the woman is at risk of going into preterm labour (as in my pregnancy with Joel).[10] It was pitting one risk against another – the risk of prematurity caused by the excess fluid versus the risk of miscarriage from sticking a needle blindly into the womb. As for antibiotics and anaesthesia during such procedures, they were not routine in medical practice until the middle of the twentieth century.

The riskiness of pushing sharp objects into a pregnant woman was well understood. In 1930s Britain, when abortion was illegal and carried a threat of life imprisonment for mother and abortionist, pregnant women wanting to miscarry inserted into their wombs slippery elm bark, crochet hooks, darning or knitting needles, hair or hat pins, wax tapers or pencils. Cheap, unqualified abortionists of the time used syringes, clay pipes and silver and glass catheters to inject noxious substances into the uterus, risking sepsis. A common medical method used to induce abortion from the 1930s until the early 1970s, soon after abortion was legalized in Britain, was a needle plunged into the amniotic sac, injecting a solution known to induce miscarriage.[11]

What changed everything was the ability to *see* into the secretive world of the unborn human baby; to know and control for the first time in history where those needles were going.

X-ray came into use at the start of the twentieth century, and for the first time there was a way to visualize a living baby in utero – confirming conditions that could only be guessed at before, like multiple pregnancies or oversized skulls – yet it could produce only a 'still' image, a snapshot. And it was far from safe. Radiological solutions were imprecisely injected into the amniotic fluid in an attempt to show the outline of the placenta in suspected cases of placenta praevia (in which the placenta covers the cervix) – but, of course, occasionally the injection sparked labour.[12]

Still, X-ray imaging in pregnancy was common in the 1950s, and in New Zealand in 1963 it was used in the first successful fetal blood transfusion, for the anaemia caused by a deadly fetal problem, rhesus disease. In 1940, it was discovered that there is another blood type as well as the blood groups identified around the turn of the twentieth century (O, A, B and AB) – we are all either rhesus positive or rhesus negative (the name rhesus comes from the rhesus monkeys used in experiments to find this new blood type). Most people are rhesus positive but about 15 per cent of British women have rhesus negative blood.[13] If a mother is rhesus negative but a father has rhesus positive blood, the child may inherit the father's blood type. And so, during childbirth, or occasionally during a first pregnancy, when the baby's blood first mixes with the mother's, a mother who is rhesus negative will be exposed to a rhesus positive baby's blood cells. When this happens, the mother's immune system is prompted to fight rhesus positive cells; in effect she becomes immunized against them. In her next pregnancy, if the baby is also rhesus positive, the mother's body will reject the baby by destroying its blood cells, leaving the baby severely anaemic in the womb – its red blood cells decreasing, the body failing to carry oxygen – and likely to die.

This is a unique disease of the fetus. Both the mother and the baby are, in themselves, healthy; there is only a problem of incompatibility – her immunity to her own baby – while the baby is in utero. After birth, blood transfusions could be done to treat the anaemia (as well as light therapy, today),[†] but if the anaemia is severe, the baby may develop hydrops fetalis and die before birth.[‡]

Albert William Liley, a pioneering New Zealand doctor – and arguably the first true fetal medic – used X-ray in 1963 to guide a transfusion needle thrust through the mother's skin and then the uterus, finally reaching into the fetus's abdomen, to give it blood to treat the anaemia. The daring procedure was highly acclaimed and repeated around the world, but it required a lot of skill and luck. It was hit and miss and sometimes the results were worse than not doing anything.[14]

Besides, by the time Liley was doing the first blood

---

† A baby with rhesus disease can develop jaundice – when the red blood cells break down, they create excessive amounts of a brownish-yellow substance called bilirubin which in turn, if untreated, can cause neurological problems. During light therapy a baby is placed under a bright lamp; their skin absorbs the light, which adds oxygen to the bilirubin so the body can break it down and get rid of it.

‡ Joel had hydrops fetalis too – but when it was discovered, tests showed I wasn't rhesus negative.

transfusions on fetuses, X-rays in pregnancy were already being recognized as a very serious danger, thanks to a brilliant Oxford University epidemiologist, Dr Alice Stewart. In 1955, she was appalled to discover that the children of those who had had prenatal X-rays were twice as likely to have developed leukaemia. Stewart published a landmark report showing that X-rays could cause radiation damage to pregnant women and their unborn children. At a time when the nuclear industry was peaking, her findings were received with outrage by doctors as well as the industry and it took until the mid- to late 1970s before the practice of prenatal X-rays finally died out. Stewart went on to become one of the twentieth century's staunchest opponents of nuclear radiation.[15]

Plunging needles and knives into pregnant women would have remained wildly dangerous had it not been for the invention of another groundbreaking technology, following the sinking of the *Titanic* in 1912. After that disaster, a new method was invented to detect icebergs and, in the First World War, to locate the position and distance of submarines. It was called sonography, and ultrasound would be the catalyst which opened up a new medical field called fetal medicine.

An X-ray captures wavelengths of light we are unable to see with our eyes; ultrasound captures sound which the human ear cannot hear. When a sound wave hits a solid object at a right angle, it is reflected back and a receiver can pick up this 'echo' and display it on a screen – sound waves bouncing off a solid organ in the body bring back a stronger echo signal, and bright white spots or lines appear on the screen, while fluid in the body appears as black space. Unhearable sound could now be *seen* – and in the 1950s, doctors started to experiment with ultrasound detectors to find breast tumours and learn about human anatomy.

Even the most experienced mother today wouldn't recognize the first ultrasound machines: they were huge contraptions like Victorian bathtubs. One, the Tomograph Pan Scanner machine of 1958, involved the subject sitting somewhat uncomfortably in a semicircular tank of degassed water, their torso to be scanned covered in plastic film.[16]

The first person to draw the parallel between the submarine in water and the fetus in its watery sac, and to carry out the first ultrasound in utero, was a quick-tempered but brilliant Scottish obstetrician gynaecologist. Tall, red-haired Ian Donald was a workaholic, fuelled by his severe rheumatic heart disease – having endured a number of mitral valve operations, every moment was precious to him.[17]

Serving in the air force in the Second World War – during which he was decorated for gallantry after rescuing injured airmen from a burning bomber plane – he had been attached to Coastal Command, where he learned to use sonar technology to try to detect submarines under water. In 1950s Glasgow, using industrial ultrasound equipment intended for detecting flaws in metal products like boilers, which he had sourced at a local factory,[18] he captured the first image of an unborn baby's head, exposed on Polaroid film attached to the display.[19] Working together with a clever young engineer called Tom Brown, he went on to invent an ultrasound machine called the Diasonograph,[20] which didn't need the patient to be suspended in water.

The very first images of babies in utero were mere snapshots showing white blurs on black screens – it was hard for Donald even to be sure which part was the placenta in a scan of a baby at thirty-four weeks' gestation, although he was able to make out the outline of the fetal head. Yet Donald saw the potential of using ultrasound to see inside the womb because ultrasound easily picked up a solid object in a liquid. A mother with polyhydramnios – too much amniotic fluid around her baby, as I had with Joel – was one of the first images Donald published: the problem of the 'enormously distended amniotic sac' bursting with fluid was relatively easy to spot. He was able to recognize the outline of twins in a vertex presentation (with their heads down) at thirty-seven weeks, but his main amazement was about a 'very interesting' case he managed to solve by ultrasound.

One of his patients had endured three months' irregular vaginal bleeding and presented with a very hard enlargement of the uterus. Having been diagnosed previously with a fibroid in her womb, she was admitted to hospital for it to be removed. But a scan showed a very different picture.

A 'mass' was in the womb – but to Donald, 'clearly a very early foetus'. He wrote: 'The result of the Aschheim-Zondek [pregnancy] test† ordered was awaited with considerable excitement since clinically the diagnosis was convincingly that of fibroid. The test was positive; and with rest in bed the patient's bleeding ceased, and she was discharged home with the pregnancy continuing. She has since been safely delivered.' [21]

It was the first time a scan showed early pregnancy, and it averted an operation that would probably have caused a miscarriage. The implications were tremendous.

---

† The early history of pregnancy tests is as bizarre as that of fetal medicine. First developed by Selmar Aschheim and Bernard Zondek in 1928, women's urine was injected into mice, rabbits and toads, which were then killed and dissected – the effect of the urine on animals' reproductive organs was different if the urine was full of pregnancy hormone. This was the standard test for pregnancy until the invention of more modern lab and then home tests in the 1960s and 1970s.

But by today's standards, the first pictures of the fetus were primitive, so fuzzy it was virtually impossible even to begin to interpret what they showed. The Diasonograph was 8 feet high and filled a third of the scanning room – earning it the nickname 'The Dinosaur'.[22]

The subjects of the earliest experiments were Donald's own gynaecological and obstetric patients at Queen Mother's Hospital, Glasgow, simply because these were the patients he had access to.[23] He even scanned his own grandchild when his daughter Caroline was pregnant. It seems there was no burning objective in doing the first scans of pregnant women – no way of predicting how big this technology could become. Fetuses in utero were just experimental subjects, along with women with ovarian cysts and cancers.

But a junior doctor, only eighteen years old at the time he started working at the Queen Mother's Hospital as a trainee obstetrician, was to take ultrasound further than anyone had dreamed possible. Stuart Campbell was in the right place at the right time, with the right techniques. He had grown up in Glasgow and, having found obstetrics his best subject at medical school, was excited to get a position working under Ian Donald, the 'number one guy' at the new hospital. Even though Donald was 'a very irascible fellow', Campbell remembers today, he was also genuine: 'a most generous and principled man'.[24]

When I met Campbell at the Royal Society of Medicine in 2017, he was eighty-one, tall and smart, still working hard – as the director of a private reproductive medicine clinic – with a down-to-earth, wry sense of humour and a taste for golf, theatre and (with our cups of tea) pain au raisin. Today Campbell is recognized as one of the pioneers of fetal medicine, but at the dawn of the 1960s, he was a young man with vision.

Donald, he remembered, 'was doing his work in this very darkened room in the ground floor, way down in the dungeon in Queen Mother's hospital, in the darkness. Nobody went down there; I was the only junior doctor who did.'

When not delivering babies, as he was employed to do, Campbell went down in his spare time and watched Donald scanning pregnant women. One day, he plucked up the courage to ask Donald: 'Can I learn how to scan?' Campbell told me, 'At that time, we were monitoring people in space, on the moon. And nobody knew anything about a fetus a couple inches below the maternal abdomen. That just fascinated me.'

Campbell set up his own clinic on Sunday mornings, again in his spare time, and worked out how to measure a baby's head accurately in the womb, allowing him to chart babies' growth through pregnancy.

The mothers must have been thrilled to get a glimpse of their babies, I said to him. 'That might have been part of it, but they wanted to be helpful, really,' corrected Campbell. 'Glasgow women are wonderful.'

No one else seemed to have much faith in what they were doing. Campbell recalled Donald showing senior physicians ultrasound images of pregnancy. 'People were actually laughing – it was *horrible*. And I thought: "How could they be so stupid? This is visionary. And they're mocking these pictures."'

Accessing a live fetus was, it seemed, a patently absurd impossibility. X-ray in pregnancy hadn't taken off in the long term – and throughout the 1960s few people believed ultrasound would, either.[25]

With the first tests for human chromosomes using amniotic fluid developed in the 1950s, the ability to test for a genetic condition in utero was launching another major chapter in fetal medicine (see chapter 6, 'Diagnosis'). Into the early 1970s, amniocentesis for genetic testing, still rare, continued to be done usually without ultrasound guidance – even though by this time it would have been technically possible. Scanning was usually only used *before* the procedure, to identify a pool of amniotic fluid.[26] But during the actual procedure when the needle went in, the scanner was (bewilderingly from today's perspective) switched off. The miscarriage rate was high when done blindly, but it was just routine at the time.[27] Amniocentesis was literally a stab in the dark.

Doctors still hadn't fully understood what scanning could do – unsurprisingly, given the crude limits of early scanning machines. But by the mid-1970s, a revolution was in full swing. As medics told engineers what they needed, engineers invented better machines, and from the middle of the decade, scanning which showed the fetus moving in 'real time' became widespread in hospitals, using small, easily movable probes. To be able to see a fetus moving in the womb had never before been possible. Campbell's eyes lit up when he told me of the world of the fetus he uncovered, his voice a scratchy Glaswegian burr. 'It's hiccupping from ten weeks. It's even opening its eyes around twenty weeks. It's making stepping movements at twelve weeks.' No one had realized any of this before.

But Campbell was about to stumble on something else big; something that would forever change the lives of children born with disabilities and, indeed, the way people think about disability. Now at Queen Charlotte's Maternity Hospital in west London, he was doing a scan of a mother-to-be on 13 March 1972 when he noticed something was very wrong with the child.

The mother had suffered for three years with infertility and wasn't having periods. She attended the hospital for fertility treatment and, in November 1971, after drug treatment, she finally ovulated. In those days, this was confirmed with a vaginal smear test rather than a scan. Her pregnancy appeared to proceed normally, until the spring day Campbell did a routine scan to check that the induced ovulation hadn't resulted in her conceiving twins, and to check the baby's measurements.

The baby's anatomy was so obviously abnormal that he couldn't miss it – it was missing part of its skull, a condition called anencephaly which is lethal at birth. Campbell told me: 'This was amazing because this was before twenty weeks and [the baby was] very small. And the pictures were black and white and grainy. But I could see that the head shape wasn't there. And I repeated it and it wasn't there.'

He repeated the scan over two weeks, 'principally to convince the patient that the finding was true'. The mother requested a termination, and with painful contractions gave birth to the fetus. The next day she went home, keen to try to get pregnant again, and the diagnosis was confirmed by the pathologist.[28] It was the first time in history that an unborn baby had been officially diagnosed with a disease by ultrasound alone.

Apart from a few anecdotal reports, it seems the idea simply had not occurred to anyone before. Campbell later wrote: 'To be honest, prenatal diagnosis of congenital abnormalities was not uppermost in my mind so it was an unexpected dilemma when I detected a case of anencephaly.' His mentor Ian Donald, an ardent Christian,[29] was 'violently' against abortion[30] and, given the reactions some parents would inevitably have on finding their baby had a serious or even deadly illness, Donald would never have pursued seeking out congenital defects in utero. But now a new world was opening up where unborn children could be routinely diagnosed with disabilities.

Who was this mother who lost her baby and how did she feel? The case report Campbell wrote at the time describes her as a twenty-five-year-old Pakistani factory worker,[31] and recorded that she was told to return for another scan when she became pregnant again and reached fourteen weeks. Today, Campbell does not remember the personal details, or whether she did go on to conceive again.

He wrote compassionately in the *Lancet* at the time, though: 'The delivery of an anencephalic infant in the 3rd [sic] trimester of pregnancy . . . is an emotionally traumatic experience for the parents . . . at present, the only available approach to the problem is to reduce distress by diagnosing the abnormality early enough for the pregnancy to be terminated.'[32]

With real-time scanning, the invasive procedure of amniocentesis was performed under ultrasound for the first time, making it much less likely to cause miscarriage.[33] Now, doctors could peer into the womb and see the mysterious baby at last. That, combined with the diagnostic breakthroughs of modern genetics and biochemical lab testing, would change everything.

Fetal medicine developed in tandem with other advances: the pill in 1960; the 1967 Abortion Act; the women's rights movement of the 1970s; fertility treatment. Women were starting to have babies later and invest everything in one or two children. New ethical questions arose. Who was the more important patient: the mother or the fetus?

In 1965, the Swedish photographer Lennart Nilsson published colour photographs of fetuses in the American magazine *Life*, causing a sensation. (They were presented as in utero photos of living babies, but they were in fact miscarried and aborted fetuses.) The magazine sold eight million copies in the first four days after publication. Nilsson's book, *A Child is Born*, was an international bestseller. His images gave the fetus an iconic position in twentieth-century public imagination.[34]

The fetus acquired celebrity status – immortalized in Stanley Kubrick's 1968 film *2001: A Space Odyssey* with its 'star child' floating in space (some of Nilsson's photographs were, in fact, sent into space with the 1970s Voyager mission,[35] presumably in case a capsule of human artefacts was ever found by aliens).

'Far from being an inert passenger in a pregnant mother, the fetus is very much in command of the pregnancy,' wrote the New Zealand fetal doctor Albert William Liley in his aptly named 1972 essay 'The Foetus as a Personality', in which he described the rich life of the developing fetus. If an unborn baby had an active life it was a patient: what rights should it have to treatment; to life? What should doctors do when they found something 'wrong'? Fetal politics – what some have called 'the cult of fetal personhood'[36] – was born, and with it a fierce abortion debate. Liley campaigned against abortion until his suicide in 1983, which some have speculated was caused by stress from his dual role as a doctor and activist for a controversial cause.[37]

*

The goal of medicine, and what is needed to establish a new branch of medicine, is treatment – the possibility of saving lives. If the 1970s was the decade when prenatal diagnosis took off, the 1980s heralded the true start of fetal medicine. With scanning only coming into routine use from the late 1970s and early 1980s, medical interest at the time focused on a different way of accessing and actually treating the mysterious world of the unborn child, using a device called a fetoscope.

By this time the junior doctor from Glasgow was a professor at London's King's College Hospital, where he was setting up the first fetal medicine unit in Britain, the Harris Birthright Centre, and a new promising young obstetrician was starting to make his mark. A junior doctor, Charles Rodeck became intrigued 'by gaining access to the fetus, which was so inaccessible,' he told me years later when we met in an anonymous room at UCH. He was now an honorary figure there, and a kindly, dapper grandfather, history buff and lover of classical and folk music who still lived in London. As a young man, he saw first-hand older doctors' scepticism about ultrasound, 'laughing at it, saying: "You don't believe those snowstorm pictures, do you?"' Stuart Campbell had proved them wrong with his diagnoses of congenital abnormalities in unborn babies. But samples of fetal blood or tissue could help doctors to make diagnoses, Rodeck knew.

At Yale University in the USA, an obstetrician called John Hobbins had started to use a strange experimental new device he called a fetoscope. Through this thin hollow cannula, a needle could be threaded into the womb under ultrasound, and a doctor could also gaze directly into the womb down the tube thanks to a fibre-optic light (in later decades, a telescopic camera also projected the close-up image of the fetus on a TV screen).

At a time when ultrasound was still in its dark ages, Rodeck initially hoped a fetoscope would allow clearer observation of the fetus. Unfortunately, 'it became pretty clear that through this very fine telescope you really couldn't see the recognized structures very well' – the image one sees through a fetoscope is too close up to get a panoramic view of the baby as was – later – easy with ultrasound. It's like looking at the surface of the moon in detail through a telescope rather than seeing the outline of the moon in the sky.

Yet a fetoscope was a way to get samples from an unborn baby. A sample of red blood cells mixed with amniotic fluid, scraped by the needle from the blood vessels on the surface of the placenta, could diagnose thalassaemia, sickle-cell disease and haemophilia, serious inherited disorders of the red blood cells. Sickle-cell disease and its more deadly cousin thalassaemia are the commonest genetic disorders in the world,[38] often affecting people from Mediterranean, African, Caribbean and Asian countries. Being a carrier of sickle cell or thalassaemia is not a problem and in fact it's believed carrying the genes offers some protection from malaria – but when two carriers have a child, the child can inherit the affected gene from both parents and become ill, needing blood transfusions throughout life. These blood diseases were not a problem in the womb – they only caused symptoms after birth. But the possibility of diagnosing them in utero – and then being able to offer mothers an abortion if they chose it – was now possible.

With a flood of immigration to Britain, many of the pregnant women local to King's College Hospital were carriers. Thalassaemia, in those days, was 'a ghastly life sentence', Rodeck observed. Some parents had more than one affected child. 'Their lives were backwards and forwards to hospital, getting transfusions every week, watching them die.' Charles Rodeck went to Yale in 1976 to learn how to use the fetoscope, and managed to smuggle the strange-looking device back through British Customs. The hope was to replicate Hobbins' ability to diagnose thalassaemia and sickle-cell disease in Britain. Neither doctor imagined that experimenting with the fetoscope would lead to being able to perform relatively safe fetal blood transfusions, for the first time in history.

They started practising with the fetoscope on pregnant women – trying to take blood cells from the surface of the placenta, as John Hobbins had done. This new procedure was so risky to the fetus that it could only be trialled with women who were having terminations – whether for 'socio-psychiatric' reasons, as Campbell recalled to me, or because of fetal abnormalities, typically a high risk of haemophilia. The women were operated on by Rodeck under general anaesthetic in an operating theatre, with Campbell operating the real-time ultrasound machine. A pregnant woman helping research before having a termination, Campbell remembered, 'sounds terrible', but 'very often gave the one bright spot to a very tragic situation for her and she could find some benefit, some altruism in it.'

During one procedure in 1977, Rodeck, 'in desperation' to get a sample, rather impulsively stuck the needle into a 'juicy' blood vessel in the fetus's umbilical cord – a spot doctors had always avoided before, for fear it could spasm and trigger miscarriage. It didn't go into spasm. For the purposes of the experiment, the fetus was fine (a termination was to follow). And the person aspirating the needle said: 'There's pure blood coming out.'[39] Rodeck realized he had discovered a way to draw pure blood from a fetus for the first time.

Previously, with the fetoscope, the blood samples from the placenta were usually a mixture of fetal blood, maternal blood and amniotic fluid. They were often difficult for laboratories to handle, but as long as there were enough fetal red cells, thalassaemia and sickle-cell disease could be diagnosed. Now that pure fetal blood could be drawn without further risk to the fetus, pure plasma (the liquid part of the blood) could be used to diagnose other conditions, like haemophilia, before birth.

One obvious target was rhesus disease, the condition the New Zealand doctor Liley had tried to treat using X-ray to guide the transfusion needle. Now, Rodeck realized, you could do a safe blood transfusion directly into the baby's circulation in utero for rhesus disease using a fetoscope and under ultrasound, and save a baby's life before birth – after which, following some exchange transfusions and treatment for jaundice, the child could grow up and lead a completely normal life. 'It was a eureka moment,' Rodeck told me. 'We had a new branch of medicine called fetal medicine.' He was 'itching' to get his hands on rhesus cases to start treatment.

A sample of blood from the fetus would also make diagnosing genetic conditions easier. As ultrasound picked up more and more babies with abnormalities, doctors started to notice that many of these babies also had genetic disorders. For instance, a baby with exomphalos – a hernia of its bowel into the umbilical cord – often also has a genetic condition. Hydrops fetalis is another case in point – many babies with hydrops turn out to have genetic disorders.

Referrals for fetoscopy sampling flooded into Rodeck and his team, becoming their main workload, but the procedure wasn't widely available to women. Doing fetoscopies was so specialist and difficult that it was only carried out in a few centres around Britain and the rest of the world.[40]

The first rhesus disease patient Rodeck was referred, a baby of twenty-four weeks' gestation, was the most affected he ever saw in his career – it had 'gross hydrops'. The doctors didn't know how much blood the fetus could take. Postnatal blood transfusions for rhesus disease were done in the neonatal unit and would take hours, with a little blood exchanged and then a little more, so as not to stress the child's circulation. Rodeck couldn't do a lengthy procedure with a fetoscope in the mother's womb – the risk of setting off labour was too great – so he had to put the fetoscope in as quickly as possible, not knowing if this in itself would kill the fetus.

He inserted the fetoscope, guided by ultrasound. It was tricky to do without hitting the baby or placenta, and with a low level of amniotic fluid because of the hydrops. If the fetoscope hit the placenta it would cause a huge gush of blood. Rodeck gazed down the tube through the cloudy, turbid amniotic fluid of later pregnancy to find the blood vessel in the umbilical cord. 'It was like looking through milk,' he told me when we met, the memory still vivid. 'The visibility was very poor but with ultrasound guidance you could see we were near the cord.' With great trepidation, he injected a small amount of blood into the blood vessel in the umbilical cord. 'It was terrifying,' Rodeck said.

The baby survived. They repeated the transfusion the following week, and the following. The hydrops got better. At thirty-two weeks the doctors decided not to push their luck and delivered the baby by caesarean section – healthy, rather to the doctors' astonishment.

After the fetoscopy technique was published, young couples from the Mediterranean, where thalassaemia was rife, started to fly to King's College Hospital for thalassaemia screening. It was very touching for Rodeck. 'These were often very poor people who'd have to sell some of their belongings to afford the fare to come over. They wanted diagnosis – they wanted to know. I felt it a terrible responsibility, because the chances of it going wrong in these early days seemed quite high, and they'd have wasted all that money and effort. They weren't forced to have prenatal diagnosis; they weren't forced to terminate, but they all did.' Today, very few babies are born with thalassaemia in developed countries because prenatal diagnosis identifies most, and parents then choose to end the pregnancies.

The possibility of fetoscopy spread around the world, reaching a small, remote town in western Australia in 1983. There, Joanne, a thirty-three-year-old mother of two, had developed rhesus antibodies during a bleed in her second pregnancy. The consequences were insignificant and the baby was fine. With a go-ahead from their doctor, Joanne and Tony embarked on their third pregnancy. By chance, Joanne came across a magazine article about Charles Rodeck saving the life of a baby with rhesus disease around this time, and thought: 'I won't need anything like that.' She threw away the magazine.

Midway through the pregnancy, though, the baby stopped growing. Rhesus anaemia was diagnosed in the nearest city, Perth, and Joanne was told her baby was going to die. After crying a lot, Joanne remembered the magazine article. Extraordinarily, her sister-in-law, a GP, had that day been donated a pile of old magazines for her practice waiting area by a patient. The two women stayed up till midnight going through the copies until they found the article.

The next day, Joanne went back to her consultant in Perth with the article, but he told her, 'It's really risky; I wouldn't recommend it. You need to accept your baby's not going to live.'

On the verge of giving up hope, another coincidence occurred. Joanne told another GP at her local practice about Charles Rodeck. It turned out that Rodeck had trained the GP's husband, also a doctor. The local doctor couple phoned Rodeck that Saturday night and Joanne got on a plane to London three days later, leaving her four- and two-year-olds on the other side of the world with her husband and mother.

The first transfusion, under local anaesthetic, was a success.

The child would have died within two weeks without it. But it wasn't easy for Joanne. At that time, fetoscopy was 'like having an operation', she told me on a long-distance call from Australia years later. Her aunt, whom she was staying with in London, wasn't allowed to be with her and hold her hand. Yet, 'The only painful thing was having to lie really still – conscious of every desire to scratch – I was lying there wishing I was anywhere but doing what I was doing.' The kindly small team did the procedure in 'the most unprepossessing room you could possibly imagine, down in the bowels of King's College Hospital. It was a bit of a shock to find it wasn't a flash environment. But I recognized the people involved were incredibly dedicated and that was what mattered.' She tried to keep herself busy afterwards, sitting in the darkness of a matinee at the cinema, crying with worry that the baby might not be kicking enough.

Two more transfusions followed, and the rest of Joanne's family flew over, but Joanne went into premature labour that Christmas Eve, at twenty-seven weeks and five days. They named the baby Charles, after Charles Rodeck. Little Charles was in hospital for five months, suffering from lung damage. When he was finally well enough to leave, still on oxygen, the Royal Air Force and the Australian government worked out a way to fly Charles to Perth with a nurse escort. A hospital paediatrician was waiting for them at the airport on arrival.

Charles remained on oxygen until he was eighteen months old and suffered from recurrent infections throughout his first five years, but Joanne worked as a developmental psychologist, and Charles had all the therapies and support he needed. Gradually his health improved, and he's now a healthy man in his thirties.

Today Joanne still thinks often of that time when she

travelled alone across the world for treatment in London. And she has stayed in touch with her doctor, Charles Rodeck. Every Christmas for thirty-five years, she has sent him a card letting him know how the child she named after him was growing up.

Fetoscopic treatment continues to be used today for treating babies in the womb – for example to fire lasers at the rogue blood vessels causing twin-to-twin transfusion syndrome. But as new, less risky techniques were developed, it became possible to get samples of fetal blood from the umbilical cord, and, later, cells from the placenta, using chorionic villus sampling. Other fetal doctors perfected blood transfusions in the womb using just an ultrasound-guided needle, which was less invasive. The demand for prenatal diagnosis grew and grew, as did the niche of open fetal surgery – fetoscopy was just the start of a new branch of medicine, that of the fetus.

Patients weren't always keen on fetal medicine. Even though Rodeck and his team could now diagnose sickle-cell anaemia in unborn children – a serious genetic disease which could affect multiple children in one family – they hardly had any referrals from the local midwives. 'It wasn't something that the local Afro-Caribbean population found acceptable,' Rodeck explained to me. 'They were very averse to intervention in pregnancy and particularly to termination; a lot were devout Christians; others just thought: "You don't mess about with pregnancy." The fetal blood sampling could only be done after sixteen weeks, so it's quite late, and they didn't want to go down the road of late termination of pregnancy.' Instead, babies continued to be born with sickle-cell disease, and mothers hoped the case would be mild and that the child would survive as long as possible.[41]

Of course, not only was diagnosis leading to termination

now possible, but so too was the potential to cure conditions. 'You might still end up terminating if that's what the parents think is the best route to take, or if you find out there is absolutely no hope for a situation,' as Rodeck said to me. But also, 'If there's a problem that's found, you don't just ignore it, you don't just get rid of it, you try and sort it out.' Doctors investigated for the first time the natural history of fetal illness, and, in America, Michael Harrison and Scott Adzick overcame seemingly impossible congenital problems with ingenious fetal surgery.

In the late 1970s and early 1980s, countries around the world started to offer ultrasound to women as part of prenatal screening. To modern mothers born before then, it's hard to grasp that their own mothers didn't get to have 'scans', let alone 3D ones. But even in 1980, fetal medicine was not widely accepted by the medical establishment. The uterus was regarded as sacrosanct, Charles Rodeck recalled to me. 'I used to get criticism from paediatricians, saying: "What are you doing meddling about with pregnancy?" People regarded it as reckless.' Many were against fetal medicine for religious reasons[42] – tampering with pregnancy was viewed in the same way as abortion (and of course many parents of babies diagnosed in utero with health conditions did, and do, abort them).

Rodeck was, as Stuart Campbell described him to me, 'an English gentleman'. But Rodeck's right-hand man, a very different character, was to become another global trailblazer for modern fetal medicine – a man Campbell described to me as 'the guru'.

The reputation of Kypros Nicolaides, the brilliant Greek who rapidly took leadership of the fetal medicine centre at King's College Hospital in south London, and is by many held to be the greatest fetal medicine specialist in the world, precedes him. 'Rough; tough', was how Stuart Campbell outlined his approach to me. Another doctor who has worked with Kypros told me (quite affectionately) how he would 'swear, shout, throw things at you'.

Mothers who have Nicolaides to thank for their babies' lives told me about long waits to see him. When I mentioned to one of his past patients that I wanted to interview Nicolaides, she wished me luck, saying: 'He's a very difficult man to get hold of. You might have success. As a patient you tend to wait about four hours for him to turn up. It's not good in that kind of situation, but he's a very busy individual. You forgive him when he arrives.'

During his operation on this mother's unborn baby, who was critically ill in the womb, Nicolaides rolled up the sleeve of his operating arm, and told her to grip it while he operated. 'I found it really comforting,' she told me. 'He's trying to make his patients feel less scared, I suppose, and give them some kind of control. He also made a joke about it, that you're squeezing his arm too hard and cutting off his blood supply. I laughed, in the middle of all that.' Having spoken to other women who have had procedures with Nicolaides, this mother heard that he told the same joke each time.

When I arrived at Nicolaides' office at the Fetal Medicine Research Unit at King's College Hospital, I was surprised. Apart from a weeping couple standing hugging at the entrance, this didn't look like part of an NHS hospital. The building – where Nicolaides has his main practice and does all his procedures – was new and gleaming. Nicolaides' sleek, minimalist office on the tranquil fifth floor, where I waited (for just twenty minutes), had panoramic views over the City and St Paul's Cathedral, a boardroom-style table and a transparent desk with metal edging, with only a couple of papers giving away that the desk was used. The chairs were white leather and more shining metal; there was modern art on the white walls. Next to the desk was a small painted ceramic, a gift from a happy former patient, which showed a grinning Nicolaides scanning a beaming hugely pregnant woman. And a glass door led to a large private roof terrace, bounteous with carefully tended greenery. A secretary brought me luxury biscuits and coffee which I drank at the boardroom table, using white coasters marked 'K' and 'N' – the doctor's initials. I was nervous; would this formidable doctor approve of me and my book?

I heard a man's voice in the corridor, and Nicolaides strode in, a robust and vigorous man in his mid-sixties, with stubble and fiery yet twinkling eyes behind glasses. The very first thing he said was: 'Let me show you my olive tree.' He led me onto his private sun terrace and showed me the baby olives he carefully tended. Then he took me to the edge of the balcony, where we gazed over the London skyline. He pointed out the old hospital opposite, where the Harris Birthright Centre began and gradually took over the top floor. In 2017, his £11 million new home for the fetal medicine unit was built, in which we now stood, funded by Nicolaides through his own charity, the Fetal Medicine Foundation, which in turn is funded through his private practice in Harley Street. The fact it doesn't look like a hospital is intentional, he told me, smiling. 'Pregnancy is not a disease. Women should not be seen in a hospital, but in an art gallery.'

Nicolaides sat down at the boardroom table for his coffee and told me how he was a 'lost' medical student at King's at the dawn of the 1980s, not sure what he would do when he graduated, when, in his last year, 'a very enthusiastic young

Scottish guy arrived as a new professor'. When he heard Stuart Campbell speak, the young student was 'overwhelmed by his enthusiasm and by the concept that you could actually look through the mother's abdomen and look at the baby for the first time in history'.

'Until then, pregnancy was a sort of mystical concept. It acquired value at the moment of birth; you could see a baby and then it was – life. Nothing much was happening before: it was happening behind an iron curtain.' Ultrasound pulled aside that curtain and being a fetal doctor was all this student wanted to do. The treatment of a fetus – how abnormalities develop, the interaction and possible conflicts between the baby and the mother, and whether it was possible to prevent problems – was, for Nicolaides, 'the philosophy of life' and 'a completely new feat of medicine'.

Rodeck and Nicolaides developed their own, different versions of Michael Harrison's shunts to drain fluid from the fetal bladder and chest in the 1980s. Had it not been for the development of a shunt treatment for fetal hydrops, my own son would certainly have died in the womb. 'I have you to thank for Joel's life,' I told Nicolaides, in awe. He lit a cigarette (hospitals are non-smoking these days, but he is not the sort of man rules like that apply to, and, of course, he did build this wing). 'I was a very junior doctor, and then suddenly within a year or two, everything we were doing was completely new. We became the leaders in the world and I was subsequently projected as one of the fathers of fetal medicine when in reality I was just a very junior trainee.' People from all over Europe and then the world started to come to the 'mecca' of fetal medicine at King's, 'the factory of ideas'.

In the early 1980s, Nicolaides worked out an easy way to identify spina bifida through ultrasound – instead of the normal 'lemon' shaped fetal head, a fetus with spina bifida has a distinctive head shape a little like a banana. And in 1991 came the step he is best known for, and which has almost certainly had the widest impact on pregnancies since the 1990s: running with the idea that large amounts of fluid beneath a baby's neck at the end of the first trimester – visible on a scan – are often a sign the baby has Down's syndrome, another chromosomal or genetic condition, or cardiac problems (see chapter 6, 'Diagnosis').

In 1992, babies with twin-to-twin transfusion syndrome (TTTS) typically died, or survived with brain damage. One night that year, a couple whose unborn twins had TTTS came to see Nicolaides. 'I was going to give them bad news and almost encourage them to have a termination because things were looking hopeless.' But then, suddenly, he thought: 'Can we actually do something about this?' He and his team ran around the hospital. 'We stole from the basement a laser machine, I had a fetoscope, and we said: "We will do a fetoscopy and try and cut the connecting blood vessels with the laser." ' It had been done before,[43] and logically the idea of the operation made sense, but he was 'extremely nervous. I didn't know what I was going to do.'

It was, he recalled, 'very, very lucky that it went well'. Today the laser surgery technique for TTTS he impulsively used that night is the standard fetal treatment around the world. Two weeks before I met him, he told me, when he had just finished the last surgery of the day, at midnight, he came to his office, and found two Italian families waiting to see him. Two sets of parents had brought beautiful identical twin girls, and handsome identical twin boys, all the children fifteen years old. In broken English, they said: 'Do you remember – you saw us years ago?' They were some of the first families he had saved with laser treatment for TTTS and had stayed in touch with each other ever since. Now they had decided to come to England and introduce the children to him. Nicolaides told me: 'It was midnight, we went out into the garden, we tried to take pictures, it was a great pleasure.'

Do baby doctors realize what a vast, lasting impact they have on the families they treat? I'm not sure. And they can't be expected to remember every life they save. But they do love to see the babies they have saved as they grow up. 'That is the biggest pleasure in life for me,' Kypros Nicolaides told me.

After speaking with me, Nicolaides invited me to follow him down the stairs to observe him operate on a mother with TTTS who had flown in from Romania for laser treatment to burn and separate the blood vessels connecting her twins and making one critically ill. I was shown into a private viewing room next to the treatment suite, with a one-way window which gave me a clear view. The mother and her friend were facing the opposite way so I could not see their faces – though they had consented to being observed through the window. It was like a small cinema – a double row of seats half filled with young doctors from all over South America who were here to observe and learn; the lights dimmed. In the viewing room we couldn't hear what was said during the operation – only watch. Still, I felt like a voyeur as I watched the nurse prep a trolley with instruments, the mother pull up her top and the friend sit close behind her, stroking her face and shoulders.

Nicolaides greeted the mother, did a quick scan and washed the cigarette smoke off his hands. The audience in the private cinema hushed abruptly as he briskly started his work, injecting local anaesthetic into one side of the pregnant belly. Just as I'd been told, he placed the woman's hand on his fore-arm. As he jabbed in the thin fetoscope, the mother's belly visibly jumped. A female doctor then fed in the long needle which fired the laser. She was clearly not doing it quite as Nicolaides would like – from the opposite side of the mother, he repeatedly pushed his trainee's hand, holding the needle, downwards to correct her angle. One false move would fire the laser at the baby.

The mother lay statue still, but I could see her breaths as her stomach rose and fell. Like setting a fire, the laser's white light burned up the blood vessels in lines, the trails of smoke like aeroplane trails.

Within half an hour of painstakingly finding and burning every rogue blood vessel, it was over. Nicolaides smiled, shook hands, and walked out of the room. Summoning me out of the viewing chamber, he was wound up. He told me how frustrated he was by his junior not getting the angle right. 'That is a very difficult procedure,' he said as he calmed down. 'I was nervous. I still have to be in control. There's fear for me . . . I don't want to hit the baby; burn the baby or the placenta. In a split second things could go disastrously wrong.'

Today, fetal medicine is a small and specialist but rapidly growing field. An expert scanner can detect many abnormalities at the end of the first trimester. More and more children are being diagnosed with medical problems in the womb, from hypoplastic left heart syndrome (in which the left side of the heart fails to develop correctly) to spina bifida to genetic conditions. And we now see more high-risk cases of twins and triplets than ever as a result of forms of assisted reproduction like IVF, and also women are giving birth in the West at a later age, which makes their pregnancies higher risk. So almost everyone today knows someone whose baby was diagnosed antenatally with some sort of complication.

Fetal doctors often appear emotionally detached to pregnant women, but although they must control their emotions to carry out procedures and deliver dire news, they have strong feelings they can't share. 'I cannot detach myself,' Nicolaides told me. 'I cannot. The concept that you get used to it . . . I feel guilty that I have not got used to it.'

And so I have come to understand that fetal medics don't see themselves, remotely, as gods.

4

Birth

'My children are born of science.'

ALLIE, NEONATAL UNIT MOTHER

Being British and easily embarrassed, I wasn't sure whether to panic and call for help. There weren't any midwives in the waiting room and the receptionists were dealing with the usual queue of patients. I felt paralysed.

It was a Monday, two and a half weeks after the shunt at the fetal medicine unit. I had returned to University College London Hospital to be registered with their midwives. We'd decided to transfer my antenatal care to this hospital because it has a high-level neonatal intensive care unit (NICU) where our son would end up anyway, even if he was born at our local hospital. And while waiting to see the midwife, I started bleeding.

My name was called and I was ushered into a room. The two midwives treated me like a normal pregnant woman. They didn't seem at all worried when I told them I was bleeding, but they listened to my baby's heartbeat to reassure me before measuring my belly and finding it was distended. The fluid had returned. The night before, Phil and I had gone to the cinema with friends and I'd found it hard to get comfortable in my seat – now I realized why.

I was admitted to the maternity ward; needles plunged steroids into my thighs to mature my baby's lungs. A belt was strapped around me to monitor for contractions, but the midwives assured me I wasn't having any. That night I hardly slept. Amid the yells of freshly born babies and the calls for midwives from the new mothers who shared the ward with me, I was wide awake, and increasingly uncomfortable. Finally, just before the dark winter dawn, the midwives turned the lights back on and fixed the monitor back around me, still assuring me I was not having contractions. I'd have a scan and see someone from the fetal medicine unit soon. Then, at 6.30 a.m., my baby kicked and water gushed over my bed.

I repressed the urge to scream and silently pressed the call button, then waited. No response. The midwives were busy down the ward; the curtains were drawn around my cubicle. I finally croaked the words 'I think I need some help', feeling silly and embarrassed. Then, louder: 'I think my waters have broken.' I was in a bay of four; I knew the other mothers just metres away in their own beds must be hearing my calls. I think one of them alerted a midwife. 'You've probably just wet yourself,' she sighed as she pulled my curtain back.

Suddenly several midwives were pushing me as fast as they could on my bed down to the labour ward. I managed to text Phil: 'Waters broke. Come', and to call my parents.

The next four hours went something like this. Waiting on my own in the delivery room while a junior doctor walked in and out, trying to scan me. A cold midwife who didn't seem to notice that I was afraid. Then, miraculously, the morning shift changed, and a new midwife took her place: a good person, who calmed me. By the time Phil and my mother ran in, the pain was getting bad. Mr Pandya stood by my bed and, still upbeat, told me confidently: 'You're going to be all right and your baby is going to be all right.'

A fair-haired, cherub-like young doctor from the neonatal unit was on call that morning. 'He's the rising star of the unit,' an admiring midwife told Phil and me. Giles Kendall busied himself in the room politely while each contraction took my breath away, interrupting our conversation in the shortening gaps in between. It was like coming in and out of conscious-ness, backing out of each snatch of rational speech with a 'Sorry, I think there's another contraction coming' every few minutes. The baby's gestation was thirty-two weeks exactly. Dr Kendall told me frankly: 'If this was a normal thirty-two-weeker, I wouldn't be worried at all, but I won't lie to you; the hydrops does make this different.' A team of people stood with him at the foot of the bed and the head midwife told me when to breathe (I had not yet started antenatal classes). A swelling, hard nut was being exploded out of me by a nut-cracker. Holding Phil's hand, I bent his fingers back so hard I nearly snapped them off. It was all too fast for an epidural. Instead they gave me paracetamol, which did nothing, then set up gas and air. I barely had the time to take a breath of it before I had to push, and then someone said they could see the baby's head.

Four hours after my waters broke, Phil and I had a baby. I knew we were supposed to hear him cry but there was silence as the doctors worked on him out of my view. My mother, Phil and I held our breaths. I never heard the little cry that should have come with my baby's first breath, but Dr Kendall soon spoke and told us our son was breathing.

The expert team in the room conveyed only quiet calmness, but according to his notes, Joel was born blue, with poor tone, making 'minimal respiratory effort', with a heart rate of forty to sixty beats per minute (normal would be three times that). He was resuscitated with oxygen fed through a tube into a face mask sealed over his nose and mouth, a doctor placing and removing a finger over a hole in the tubing to deliver pushes of air, until his colour, tone and heart rate improved.

But I didn't know any of this. For a split second they laid the baby I'd pushed out on my belly. I saw a flash of brown hair and intense blue eyes. Then he and the doctors were gone.

Across the corridor in intensive care, doctors pushed a tube into Joel's airways, attached to a ventilator machine that breathed for him. A high thrust of oxygen was dialled down as he stabilized. He was given two doses of cold, slippery surfactant, to coat the lining of his airways so he could breathe.

I had no idea what was happening on the other side of the building. The adrenaline of birth left me elated. I had experienced it moment to moment, and that strange alive feeling continued for a while. My delivery had been relatively quick and easy – 'textbook', the midwife told her student. There wasn't mental space to take in where my baby had gone; he was just that glimpse of brown hair and blue eyes. Even though I knew our child must be critically ill, I let myself feel the sparkling pride and joy any new mother feels. When the placenta came, and the doctor found a little tear that needed stitching up, I barely noticed. The staff melted away; I had a shower; ate coffee and toast, still on my hospital bed in the delivery room. My father arrived, his normally staunch eyes wet with tears.

Dr Kendall came back and told us our son was stabilized on a ventilator. He gave Phil and me two photographs the doctors had taken just before they put the tube down his throat so that we would have a picture of him looking like a normal baby, wearing a nappy and a little woollen hat to keep him warm. It surprised me that with all the technology available, a woolly hat and nappy were still priorities. In the pictures, I saw a lost-looking person whose eyes were open; the camera had frozen him mid-movement, perhaps mid-cry. He looked chubby, with colour in his cheeks (an illusion: his high colour was jaundice, and his thin face and body were swollen with the fluid of hydrops). That image was all I had of him. We walked up to the maternity ward to wait for more news. I was per-fectly well and felt full of life in an unreal, dream-like way. The baby wasn't yet a person to me: I didn't know him, I'd barely met him. I hadn't had the chance to count his fingers and toes or gaze into his eyes or touch him with my hands.

If I'd known, that afternoon, that I was allowed to visit the neonatal unit at any time of day or night and do those things, I would have. But I assumed I wasn't allowed to visit the baby. It was almost too much to take in that my son, my actual son, was just one floor below.

That evening, after Phil and our families went home, a mid-wife told me I had a slight fever. 'If you really want to go down to the neonatal unit, you can, but perhaps you have an infec-tion and should wait,' she said. That's when I started to worry. I felt perfectly healthy, but the idea that I might be carrying an infection which I could pass to my baby made me too afraid to see him. Instead I lay on my bed, wondering how I would know that I was well enough to meet him the next day.

Beside my bed in the room was a double crib – the twins of the previous mother in the room had slept there beside her. I put my photographs of Joel in the empty crib and tried not to feel like a freak of nature. In the night, I woke freezing cold and walked down the corridor hearing the squeals of newborns all around me. I asked a midwife for an extra blanket, but she told me there was none.

*

Six years after Joel's life was saved at birth, I went back to the neonatal unit at UCH when researching this book. As with the fetal medicine unit there, I felt pulled back. I wanted to understand what had happened there – and this time to understand the doctors' and nurses' view. Resuscitation is not something a NICU mother would usually ever watch. It happens immediately after a baby is born, before she has even delivered the placenta. Or if a baby in a ward suddenly needs to be resuscitated, all parents would be asked to leave the room. So it was something I had never observed, but I felt I needed to see it.

The neonatal unit was in a heightened state one Wednesday morning, because triplets were to be delivered, two of whom had twin-to-twin transfusion syndrome. By the time they were referred to the fetal medicine unit, one triplet had died; now the other two were to arrive via C-section, only thirty weeks old. I stood in the small resuscitation room which adjoins the labour ward's operating theatre, watching as nurses and doctors set everything up: two incubators, labelled 'twin 1' and 'twin 2'; a trolley for each laid out with tracheal tubes and sterile scissors; and the exact amounts of medicines each twin would need, calculated and written on a whiteboard.

Everyone was businesslike; not overtly anxious but highly focused with the tension of awaiting these babies – everything was ready for the moment of their birth. From the roles each member of the team would play to the optimal pressure levels pre-set on the ventilators to the position of the oxygen masks, heart rate stickers and little woollen hats by the nest of towels in each incubator – everything was calculated, adjusted, checked and rechecked as the minutes ticked by. The neonatal team don't always get the time to prepare like this – if a baby is born suddenly – but with this planned C-section, they had a chance to put everything perfectly in place.

The sequence they would perform is called ABC – Airway, Breathing, Circulation. A, the doctor has to position the airway so the baby can get oxygen in and carbon dioxide out. B, the doctor breathes for the baby, delivering oxygen to the lungs through a face mask. A plus B should result in C. It has to be done properly. If you don't use enough pressure to open the lungs, the circulation doesn't kick in. Or if you make the technical error of inserting the ventilator tube into the oesophagus instead of the trachea, the baby won't respond to resuscitation and could die.

One of Joel's main neonatal consultants was a little, bird-like woman, a mother of grown-up children herself with a love of babies, called Judith Meek. Now I followed her as she called the team together for a briefing. As a patient's mother I'd seen her as maternal, even grandmotherly, a keeper of strange witchy medical magic; now I saw her tough and ice-cool, her long brown hair tied back like a schoolgirl. A resuscitation, she later told me, is acutely stressful for her. There were two nurses and two doctors for each baby, in plastic gloves and surgical hats, as well as herself. She didn't expect to have to do much, she told me – she'd expect two registrars to be able to cope with two thirty-weekers, and they might not even need ventilation – but she would be right there if needed: 'You just never know.' Standing in the corner, trying to keep out of everyone's way, I could feel the anxiety in the air.

One nurse wondered aloud about how it must feel to have cold surfactant thrust into one's lungs . . . like being suffocated underwater, she imagined. Each tiny vial of the stuff costs thousands.

Suddenly a nurse monitoring the situation in theatre called out: 'Twin one is coming now. Its head is out.' A few seconds later: 'It's not vigorous. No crying.' There was a moment of shock before someone realized aloud: 'That's the deceased one.' Our two expected babies were still alive.

Minutes later, a nurse rushed into the room holding the first live baby in a towel, cut straight from the mother's womb. He was placed in the incubator nearest me; the size of an A4 piece of paper, his skin dusky (in fact, blue with lack of oxygen). The senior house officer (SHO), a straightforward, professional thirty-eight-year-old mother who looked like just the sort of person you would want to save your life, fitted the face mask attached to the ventilator over him and with her finger covered and uncovered the little hole, like playing a wind instrument, to push oxygen puffs to his nose and mouth. The monitor showed his oxygen saturation level was only at 46 per cent. They needed to get it up to the eighties and nineties, fast, if he was not to be deprived of oxygen, which can cause brain damage. An adult suffering a cardiac arrest can survive for three minutes without oxygen before brain injury starts, but a baby can cope with up to ten minutes of acute oxygen deprivation without brain damage. Ten minutes ticks by very quickly in the resuscitation room.

Working at speed, the SHO inserted a metal laryngoscope into the baby's throat to open it up. His tiny face was almost obscured by the large instrument forcing his mouth wide open. They suctioned his lungs with a tube to get rid of gunk, then the doctor fed down a tube into his trachea.

I was ready to breathe with relief but the baby's saturation had dropped to 29 per cent. His heart rate was slow – the doctor leaned over him, listening with her stethoscope. Judith Meek stepped in – 'Try another tube,' she said. As they struggled to get a new tube down his airways, saturation dropped again – to just 13. The senior house officer couldn't hear a heart rate. But Dr Meek was calm. She pointed out his eyes were open. They tried another tube. 'Take your time,' Judith said. 'Don't rush.' Unable to get a tube in, the doctors placed the face mask on again. The baby was actually trying to breathe. His saturation climbed within minutes to 46, 83, 87, 91, 94, 96, 97. His skin was now pink. I heard tiny whirrs and bleats, his helpless cries – and watched his spindly arms batting at the hands all over him. Above all, this was a little person. There was something age-old in this child's eyes. He was not an alien or a doll; he was a human being. Even a little like an elderly one rather than a young one. He had the same concerned 'Where am I?' look one sees in a very old man's eyes.

Now he needed surfactant. They managed to insert the tube easily this time, with the doctor hand-puffing air through again, and the surfactant was syringed in. All this time, the other team had been working on the second twin, and he, too, was stable now. Judith put her head around the door of the theatre and gave them a thumbs-up. Ever conscious of the parents' experience, she went outside to find the father – but it turned out the mother had sent him home because he was so stressed.

The little boys were wheeled into the intensive care nursery, towels wrapped over them to keep them warm, and hooked up to ventilators side by side. The first baby, who I saw resuscitated, was now weighed and nappied, swabbed for infections, his temperature taken. But his ordeal was not over yet. Now they would fit a cannula to take blood for tests and, through this line, give him antibiotics, and morphine for the pain of being ventilated. The SHO turned on a bright light over his incubator, found a vein in his hand and pricked in a needle for the cannula. I was standing on the other side of the incubator and I saw the baby's eyes were screwed shut, tears in the corners; his legs flexed like a frog's; his mouth hanging open. 'Hey,' I said to him softly, crying myself. 'It's gonna be OK. You're going to see Mummy soon.'

His eyes opened, widened and gazed directly at me. He looked shocked, exhausted, disbelieving. Again, like an old man. He had the finest doctors and nurses all around him, but he seemed so alone. What must he think of this world into which he had been born, and separated from his mother and his siblings? Nothing could be further from the experience of a healthy baby, who is lifted into his mother's arms after birth and who suckles and cuddles close to her safe, familiar body throughout his first hours. I was not allowed to open the porthole; he'd get cold – and perhaps he couldn't really hear me. Next he would be fitted with a nasogastric tube for feeding. The baby's skin was fuzzy; his arm as thin as unpadded, folded velvet.

It was 2.40 p.m., an hour and a half after his birth and the adrenaline in the unit was returning to its normal, averagely high levels. The nurses and doctors told one another they really should go and eat some lunch. 'Can you relax now?' I asked Judith. 'No,' she said, walking briskly away down the corridor. 'It's only a matter of time until the next emergency.' And for these triplets-turned-twins, this was just the start of a long journey in hospital.

*

The common methods of resuscitating a premature baby, according to one early British obstetrician in the 1750s, included whipping, applying brandy and holding an onion at a baby's nostrils.[1] The idea of being able to resuscitate and keep alive premature and sick babies, which we take for granted now, is a new one. For the vast majority of human history, there was no treatment, no type of hospital, no medical field for these babies. The care of newborns, let alone sick newborns, was traditionally left to mothers rather than doctors – and to luck.[2]

One of the first and most important realizations that got us where we are today was that premature babies need to be kept warm. We think of incubators as high-tech and modern, but the American father of neonatology, Julius Hess, who started the first American premature baby unit in 1920s Chicago, speculated that the Egyptians might have applied the principles of hatching hens' eggs in a warm incubator to human newborns – although he could find no evidence of this.

The care and treatment of premature and sick babies started in earnest in nineteenth-century France. The first incubator is usually traced back to 1857, when a Professor Denuce of Bordeaux devised a 'zinc cradle'. It was, in effect, a cot wrapped in insulating wool, suspended over a tub of hot water.[3]

It was a trip to the Paris zoo in 1878 that led to the modern incubator. The story goes that the pioneering French obstetrician Stéphane Tarnier had a eureka moment when he saw the zoo's incubators for the eggs of exotic birds.[4] By 1880 he had invented a closed incubator inspired by the kind used to hatch hens' eggs. It was built for him by none other than the director of the Paris zoo and could hold several babies at one time.[5] In early models, the baby lay on a mattress in a wooden box, heated from below with metal or stone hot-water bottles. A little chimney above the baby's head let the hot air flow through the contraption, and large panes of glass over the top and sides allowed doctors to observe the child closely.[6]

Preterm babies at the turn of the twentieth century were medically called 'weaklings'. The idea of focusing on infants' welfare seemed, to the leading obstetrician of the day, Tarnier's former intern Pierre Budin, revolutionary. Until his era, medical attention had concentrated on the life and death of the mother; doctors, he wrote, 'scare spared a thought for the infant'. But as understanding of antiseptic procedures grew, the obstetrician was 'freed from anxiety as to the fate of the mother' and 'could now devote his attention to the needs of the infant'.[7] With his Paris clinic systematically keeping premature babies warm and well fed with wet nurses' milk, Budin made the 'discovery', as one other doctor of the time put it, 'that we need not let infants die in the numbers that are our reproach – that an arrest can be, and has been put, on the wastage of infant life'. Another commentator hailed Budin as 'the means of saving a battalion from the slaughter-field of infancy'.[8]

In one of the most bizarre chapters in the history of neonatology, premature babies in incubators were put on public exhibition throughout the early twentieth century. A Prussian-Jewish immigrant, Martin Couney, started this strange form of entertainment at Earls Court in London in 1897, drawing thousands of visitors. He then emigrated to America and his 'Baby Incubators' exhibition became one of the most popular attractions at Coney Island amusement park for forty years. The babies in their incubators were cared for by a team of doctors and nurses. Members of the public paid 25 cents to see them from behind a guardrail – the money paid for the babies' treatment. Couney was, says his biographer Claire Prentice, 'shunned by the medical establishment, and condemned by many as a self-publicist and charlatan. But to the parents of the children he saved, and to the millions of people who flocked to see his show, he was a miracle worker.'[9]

By the 1920s, all kinds of incubator designs were in use around the world – the inventive Julius Hess even fashioned a transportation incubator crossed with a doctor's bag, designed to keep a baby warm if born prematurely outside the hospital. From the outside it looked like any doctor's attaché case, but a false bottom hid a compartment for hot-water bottles and the baby fitted in the main part of the bag. Half-inch holes beneath the bag's handle allowed for ventilation.[10]

Meanwhile in Britain, a remarkable woman decided to attack a parlous rate of mortality among premature babies and stuck to her task throughout the privations of wartime. A vicar's daughter, Dr Victoria Mary Crosse founded the first premature baby unit in Britain in 1931, in the grounds of one of Birmingham's maternity homes, with only ten spaces for infants. Her methods – 'careful attention to detail, unremitting oversight on the part of the medical officer and the devotion of a highly skilled nursing staff' – established the rigorous principles of neonatal care which continue to the present day.

The neonatal ward of the mid-1940s was rather different from today. In America, heated 'electric incubators' were used to try to stabilize babies' temperatures and surround them with oxygen (it was only understood later that overexposure to oxygen caused blindness), but as Crosse tartly wrote, 'a far simpler plan has proved successful in Birmingham. Instead of incubators, ordinary wicker washing-baskets are used.' Hot-water bottles wrapped in flannel or blankets were her solution, or even an electric blanket 'placed under the infant, well covered with mackintosh sheeting and several layers of blanket'.

Visiting doctors and nurses would be admitted only occasionally and if they were wearing masks and gowns. Parents were not admitted to the ward as a matter of course and had to content themselves with seeing their babies through a 'viewing window' or glass panel in the door or wall.

Victoria Mary Crosse understood premature babies often suffered from bleeding in the brain, and those born at low weights struggled to breathe because of poorly developed and weak lungs. She insisted babies were exposed to ultra-violet light regularly to counteract anaemia; their eyes protected with small goggles or a towel – a practice that continues today to treat jaundice. But other methods were somewhat different back then. If a baby's oxygen level plummeted – today called 'desaturation' – turning a premature child 'blue', she recommended administering 1–5 millilitres of brandy by mouth or a minuscule injection of strychnine. And she added: 'Expansion of the lungs can be encouraged by making the infant cry at regular intervals,' though she clarified, 'Any means used to achieve this end must be gentle, and such a procedure as slapping is not to be advocated. Mustard baths, which have been suggested for mild cases, should not be used because of the amount of handling entailed.' Oxygen was delivered to very small babies through oxygen beds, tents or hoods, or a soft rubber mask placed over the nose and mouth.[11]

Units even as advanced as this were few and far between. At University College London Hospital, there was no premature baby unit as such in the 1940s – only a side office kept by a nurse called Sister Edwards.[12] A young house officer training at the hospital, Herbert Barrie, who went on to become a leading neonatologist, remembered it near the end of his life as 'a linen cupboard', explaining: 'If she thought a baby needed special care, that is where the baby went.' Sister Edwards, he said, didn't allow other medical staff to go near this cupboard, which in those primitive days, Barrie joked, 'was probably a good thing'.[13]

Still, the blossoming idea of detailed clinical observations of premature babies – later a crucial part of what came to be called 'intensive care' – allowed doctors to understand for the first time the specific problems of these patients. One was neonatal jaundice; another was the deadly inability of premature lungs to breathe, finally given a name: respiratory distress syndrome (RDS). The idea of resuscitating babies who could not breathe began to take off. Since the early 1800s, doctors had tried to pump air into sick babies' lungs through a syringe or bag,[14] but it isn't so easy to kick-start premature lungs and keep them breathing. Now, in the second quarter of the twentieth century, came more sophisticated mechanical 'ventilators' or breathing machines.

The first machines, also known as iron lungs, used 'negative pressure'. A polio patient whose breathing muscles were paralysed lay in an airtight chamber. A pump sucked the air out of the chamber, and the low pressure around the patient's chest made their lungs expand, forcing an in-breath. In the 1940s and 1950s, 'positive pressure' ventilation took over – instead of air being pumped *out*, it was pumped *in* at intervals into the patient's lungs through a face mask or a tube into the throat.

Having noticed the remarkable effects of positive pressure ventilation, doctors realized this technique could help babies with RDS, too. Virginia Apgar, a professor of anaesthesiology at Columbia University in New York (famous for inventing the Apgar scale which grades from one to ten how healthy a newborn is within their first moments), started to resuscitate babies by delivering oxygen to them through a rubber tube into their trachea.

At the end of the 1950s, Herbert Barrie introduced this basic form of ventilation at St Thomas's Hospital in London. But he soon discovered that after some babies were resuscitated, they stopped breathing again as soon as the ventilation stopped. The most premature babies often just could not start to breathe on their own. The problem was how to go on ventilating them, potentially for days on end. At this point, there were no reliable mechanical ventilators – the positive pressure puffs of oxygen the ventilator delivered came from a human finger covering and uncovering an opening on the tube into the trachea. 'Fortunately, we had an endless supply of immensely fit medical students at St Thomas' and we put them to work, which they did willingly,' Barrie later said. 'They sat there for hours finger-ventilating.'[15] Yet it wasn't enough; these tiniest-ever hospital patients soon died.

Finally, in 1963, a new ventilator gave Barrie his first survivor from RDS. The 'fearfully complicated' Bird respirator – invented by an aviator inspired by high-altitude breathing technology developed by the Germans in the Second World War – had been developed not to help premature babies breathe, but adults having heart surgery, another new field that was growing faster and was better funded than neonatology.

Barrie also realized that the rubber tubes used for resuscitation were not up to the job. They caused intense irritation to a baby's larynx after only a few hours of use. So he switched to plastic tubes – but this brought up a new question: whether and how to sterilize them. When heated, the plastic tubes simply melted. Barrie fashioned his own tubes and hid them in small paper packets in the hospital's radiotherapy department, hoping the radiation would sterilize them. Eventually manufacturers started to make single-use sterile plastic tubes of the kind hospitals use today.

The British 'father of neonatology', credited with working out how to save premature babies without disabling them, was a 1952 Olympic fencer turned paediatrician, Osmund Reynolds. This calm, shy man – everyone called him Os – always seemed to know what to do; his babies were considered safe. Tall and athletic, Os joked in later life that he may not have been the best student of physiology, but he had been busy winning a team bronze medal for fencing at the 1955 world championships. The truth was that he was very clever.

Understanding that no two babies are the same, for Os, ventilating was never a case of blindly following a guideline for a typical baby. Instead, he considered the individual biology of each baby and worked out exactly what they needed on any particular day. He also cared about what happened to children as they grew older – and was among the first neonatologists to do follow-ups. At a time when ventilated babies were routinely disabled and people questioned why anyone should bother saving them, Os believed that if doctors could manage related issues like low blood sugar and jaundice, these children could develop healthily.[16] His brilliance wasn't limited to medical nous – it was also in how he ran the unit. He recognized that neonatal nurses were just as important as the doctors. The reliance placed on nurses was reflected in the procedure book at University College Hospital. The first page just said, 'Sister knows it all'.[17] Together with a legendary, motherly nurse called Anthea Blake, who had a solution to any problem, would intubate babies herself when necessary, and even designed the knitted hats prem babies wore, Os founded the premature and sick baby charity Bliss.[18]

Still, most babies continued to die from RDS[19] until a breakthrough came. The main reason why the survival rate was so low, it emerged, was because these babies lacked surfactant. Lungs are made up of little stretchy sacs called alveoli. Oxygen diffuses into the bloodstream through these sacs' outer membranes, and when the sacs inflate, more oxygen can be absorbed because the sacs have a greater surface area. In the late 1950s, scientists discovered that a liquid compound of fat and protein which develops naturally in term babies in time for birth, called surfactant – slimy and slippery, with the texture of shampoo – makes it easier for the alveoli to inflate and stay inflated. Newborn lungs are like balloons – increasingly fragile the more tautly they are inflated. Surfactant is a coating which stops those little balloons deflating. Now, Mary Ellen Avery, a Harvard Medical School researcher, showed that premature babies' immature lungs lacked surfactant, so their lungs couldn't expand. Due to the inflammation of the alveoli when breathing without surfactant, a glassy membrane called hyaline forms in the air sacs, making it hard for them to take in oxygen. Babies' breathing became laboured, fast and shallow as the air sacs remained collapsed.

Babies whose lungs were slightly more mature had enough surfactant for their lungs to expand with air and so they could breathe on their own at birth. Even if they then needed to be ventilated, they usually survived. But those whose lungs didn't expand naturally, who were too premature to have developed the surfactant to breathe by themselves initially, almost all died despite ventilation forcing their lungs to take in air.[20] President John F. Kennedy and his wife Jackie's son, Patrick Bouvier, born only five-and-a-half weeks premature at a relatively high weight in 1963,[21] was one of those whose lives could not be saved. It took decades – until the 1980s – for scientists to develop a successful replacement surfactant – a medicine that could be delivered to the baby's lungs within seconds by syringing it through an endotracheal tube.[22]

Gradually, hospitals started to establish intensive care units to treat newborns using ventilators, intravenous fluids and round-the-clock nursing. But, as with fetal medicine, neonatology was woefully underfunded. As late as 1980, there were still only twelve neonatal consultant posts in the whole of Britain.[23] It was only in the 1980s that staff numbers improved – just in time to offer intensive care to a growing group of children. Not only was fetal medicine saving lives, but thanks to advancing fertility treatments there were growing numbers of multiple pregnancies[24] – which have a higher risk of premature birth. Premature babies who would not have been considered viable were starting to survive regularly, thanks to developing ventilation and CPAP (a less invasive breathing machine), the widespread introduction of surfactant, and total parenteral nutrition, which delivers through an intravenous drip to babies the fluids and nutrients they need at a time when their stomachs cannot yet process milk.

Attention in the 1970s and 1980s turned to understanding the brain haemorrhages and lesions caused to some premature babies by being ventilated or starved of oxygen at birth – now doctors could see the neurological damage using newly developing imaging techniques.[25] Os Reynolds became best known for innovating the cooling of babies, which is now a standard treatment to reduce brain damage. Another colossal leap forward came in the mid-1990s, with mothers at risk of preterm labour receiving steroid injections to mature unborn babies' lungs.[26]

Doctors could now save lives, but were those lives going to be worth living? For years there had been tensions over – as one doctor summarized – what 'those immoral, obsessed, over-treating blighters in the neonatal unit are up to over-treating these infants, not letting them die in peace, and making sure they end up handicapped'.[27]

Between 2004 and 2017 alone, the number of children in Britain with complex needs rose by more than 50 per cent.[28] The lives of more and more people with congenital disabilities are being saved. In addition, the medical treatment sick babies experience can save their lives but can also cause physical and neurodevelopmental disabilities. Arguably as a result of this medical revolution, society has had to become more accepting of disability.

Some say the watershed occurred in April 1982 with the sad case of a baby boy who became known as Baby Doe and a symbol for all children born with disabilities.[29] A child was born in Bloomington, Indiana. He was blue and quickly diagnosed with Down's syndrome, as well as a serious gut obstruction called oesophageal atresia, combined with tracheo-oesophageal fistula, an abnormal connection between the trachea and oesophagus. The obstetrician reportedly described the child to his parents as a 'blob' and said he would be severely retarded. He advised them not to consent to an abdominal operation on offer, which would have very probably saved his life. The alternative to treatment was to let the baby die of pneumonia, which would be the natural result of his oesopha-geal malfunction. After thirty minutes' discussion the parents agreed the baby should be left to die.

Baby Doe could have been sent for surgery and fed with intravenous fluids. But the morning after his birth, the obstet-rician told the nurses in the neonatal unit not to feed him intravenously and instead said they could feed him orally, even though he would choke, especially as he was also kept sedated – for no medical reason. Other doctors disagreed with the decision not to give life-giving treatment and the nurses flat-out refused to follow the instructions they had been given. So Baby Doe was moved to a private room. Several families asked to adopt Baby Doe to save his life, but his own parents refused. Lawyers tried to fight the parents' decision but were unsuccessful.

After several days, Baby Doe was spitting blood, parched and weak. Six days after his birth, he died. His birth certificate disingenuously said he had died of multiple congenital birth defects. The public outcry about the case was so strong that America passed a new law, stating that hospitals and doctors must not withhold treatment from disabled infants.

And so, with advances in medicine, public opinion shifted and sick newborns were protected. In believing that babies' lives might against all the visible odds turn out to be worth saving, the early baby doctors had an extraordinary faith.

In practice, though, giving life-saving treatment to a sick baby still remains a judgement call for doctors and parents. If Baby Doe was born today, he would never be left to die, because his disabilities would not be considered major, but other newborn babies are now considered so seriously ill that the quality of their life – and the act of resuscitation – comes into question. All that has really changed is the limit of what medicine can do. Viability is the cut-off point at which a baby is given medical treatment; it is the age at which abortions are no longer permitted in Britain, except for medical reasons. By the 1980s, babies born under twenty-eight weeks were thought viable. (Compare that to just a few decades earlier: 97 per cent of the premature babies born at under twenty-eight weeks' gestation and treated in Victoria Mary Crosse's premature baby unit between 1931 and 1943 died.)[30]

By the mid-1990s, a baby born at twenty-four weeks had a reasonable chance of survival; twenty-four weeks became the moment at which neonatologists considered a baby 'viable'. Over the years since then, that threshold has been pushed further back, but more slowly.

The youngest baby ever to survive, James Elgin Gill, was born at twenty-one weeks and five days, in 1987, in Ottawa, Canada. It's interesting that this landmark was reached when neonatal medicine was still in its infancy; you might wonder why more babies this premature or even more premature are not routinely saved thirty years later. It is in fact possible to save the lives of twenty-two-weekers at the current frontier, but almost all babies born so early have disabilities, to an extent that it's widely considered by the medical profession that they don't have a good quality of life.

The current survival rate for twenty-three-weekers is now 60–65 per cent.[31] And on whether to resuscitate a twenty-three-weeker, medical opinion is divided. 'I've seen some who are fine, but there are lots who aren't, and you can't predict it at the time you're resuscitating them,' one consultant paediatrician at a British hospital told me. 'It's a value judgement on what makes a life worth living.' The parents typically don't know what to think either when it comes to this 'grey zone', she has found.

Of course, dating babies' gestational age based on their scan measurements and the date of a last missed period is often vague even today, and it could well be that a baby like James Elgin Gill, whose age was thought to be twenty-one weeks and five days, was actually nearer twenty-three weeks. Joel was technically born at thirty-two weeks because of the dates given to us at scans, but I had been monitoring my ovulation and I believe his actual age at birth was thirty-one weeks. Many neonatologists prefer to make a decision to resuscitate based on a baby's weight instead of their age. If they are more than 500 grams, they are in with a good chance. Twenty-three-weekers who weigh 500 grams are now often given medical treatment; even twenty-two-weekers at a relatively big weight.

Giving birth to a baby on the threshold of viability is the sharp end of premature birth. Eve, an occupational therapist and family psychotherapist who has always struck me with her sure-minded, protective motherliness, is a friend I made later, when we got chatting in a hospital outpatient waiting room with our babies. Forty-one-year-old Eve was twenty-one weeks pregnant when she started bleeding fresh, red blood. She and her husband Charlie, an artist and carpenter, had fallen pregnant with non-identical twins in their second round of IVF, after the first cycle ended in a traumatic missed miscarriage at eleven weeks. Because of their fertility treatments, their private clinic was scanning Eve regularly, and early on, it was clear that one embryo was lagging behind the other. At twelve weeks, the fetus didn't appear to be developing normally – there was evidence of acrania, a lethal condition where the skull does not form fully, and the child also had a heart defect and was too small – the prognosis of acrania alone was so hopeless that the couple didn't feel it necessary to ask what the heart problem was. Their baby wouldn't live after birth.

Eve and Charlie had decided to continue with their pregnancy. Preparing themselves to say goodbye to the dying twin after birth was the choice they felt they had to take, because 'reducing' the pregnancy posed a greater risk to their healthy baby. But, at her regular scans, the naturally confident Eve couldn't look at the screen. The healthy twin was a boy they named Noah; the twin who wasn't viable was a girl. They called her Amber. Eve already knew, thanks to her time in the fetal medicine unit, that Amber had no chance of survival after birth. All their hopes were hanging on Noah surviving.

Now at twenty-one weeks, rushing with Charlie to hospital, Eve was admitted to an antenatal ward which doubled as the postnatal ward. Many British hospitals have the same set-up, but for mothers with ill babies, having to share a room with loud newborns and their proud mothers is a kind of hell, as I also discovered. Eve didn't know what was happening and was seen only by junior doctors and midwives. After a week, she was relieved to be moved to a side room and was told when she stopped bleeding, she could go home. Then, at twenty-three weeks and one day, the severe pains started.

This being by far the furthest she had ever reached in a pregnancy before, and yet with no antenatal classes because she was only halfway through her pregnancy, Eve didn't realize she was going into labour – a miscarriage prompted by Amber's unfinished skull, and brain and heart defects. Because she had not passed the twenty-four-week viability threshold, she hadn't been offered steroids – the injection which matures the lungs of an unborn baby at risk of premature birth. The midwives told her: 'It's nothing' for twenty-four hours before someone examined her and announced: 'You're three centimetres dilated.'

Panicking midwives wheeled her at speed to the labour ward.

'You're having a miscarriage,' the obstetrician said.

'No,' said Eve, a strange adrenaline coursing through her. 'I'm having my babies.'

Eve is the sort of woman who is very secure with herself; she knows her own mind. The midwife in the labour ward gave the doctor a look which Eve translated as 'Shit, this mother doesn't understand.'

The obstetrician called the neonatologists. Suddenly everything changed. The senior neonatologist sat on Eve's bed and held her hand. She felt soothed by his soft, warm but clear manner. 'You're going to have to make a very difficult decision,' he told her. 'You're going to have to decide whether I can make the call, when the baby is born, whether to resuscitate him or not.' In between contractions, Eve phoned her friend's husband, a paediatrician.

'What would you do in my situation?' she asked him.

'I'd give him a cuddle and say goodbye,' her friend said.

With her husband and mother by her side and some gas and air, Eve gave birth to Amber, and then Noah.

Noah weighed 670 grams – minute, but a good weight for a twenty-three-weeker. Incredibly, he gasped and cried almost immediately. He was so young that his hair didn't yet have pigment – it was white. He was intubated, placed into a plastic bag to keep him warm and rushed to neonatal intensive care.

Amber had a heartbeat right up until she was born, but died immediately at birth.

The next morning, a nurse asked if Eve wanted to see and hold Amber. Eve wasn't sure, but, reassured it would be all right, Amber was wrapped in a blanket, so Eve could only see her face, hands and feet. She was tiny; only 360 grams. And she looked beautiful.

Eve's daughter died, but her son Noah took that critical first breath.

Despite the gravity of her situation, in the months to come, Eve would refuse to drop the optimism which had carried her through birth. It was a kind of madness, she has told me, but her intense hope, her denial of the touch-and-go reality facing her son who was born too young to be considered viable, was an unconscious protection instinct.

Eve had known since pregnancy that her daughter could not survive, so she had come to terms with having one baby, not two. And when it came to Noah, she was full of hope and did not have thoughts of him dying.

Seven years later, when I completed my interviews with her for this book, Eve told me she keeps her daughter's ashes in her drawer at home. She has never opened the box. 'I'm terrified of opening the box – I'm just terrified there'll be so few ashes because she was so tiny, so I just can't open the box yet,' she told me.

'Do you think you will one day?' I asked her.

She said, 'I don't know. I really don't know.'

Arranging a funeral for one baby while the other was critically ill felt 'surreal'. When you're so close to your baby's death day after day, it becomes hard to know what is normal, what is real, any more. Eve once reflected to me, 'I went a bit mad.' It was a useful, functional kind of madness, an almost irrational optimism that started with telling the labour ward staff she wasn't miscarrying but delivering, and allowed her to continue walking and talking each day, having buried one twin while the other wavered on the brink of existence.

And her optimism would pay off. With love, and the neonatologists' work over the months to come, Noah would live, and thrive.

5

Intensive Care

'The next few months are going to be a rollercoaster.'

NEONATAL INTENSIVE CARE UNIT NURSE

The first thing you see is the yellow line on the floor. That line, next to the row of washbasins in the waiting room, marks where the outside world ends, and a new world begins.

You do not just cross the yellow line.

Due to the risk of infection, only mothers, fathers and grandparents are allowed to cross the line in winter; aunts and uncles may get occasional permission from the consultant. In summer, babies' siblings are allowed over the line, and the odd family friend.

But even then, no one crosses the line until they have thoroughly washed and sanitized their hands – indeed, not just the hands, but the forearms up to the elbows. It's a many-stage procedure, itemized on illustrated posters above each washbasin. First, roll up your sleeves to above the elbow. Place hands under the automatic sensor to turn on the warm water and wet them. Use the touch-free soap dispenser to place a dose of soap onto cupped hands. Rub hands palm to palm. Right palm over the back of the other hand with interlaced fingers and vice versa. Palm to palm with fingers interlaced. Back of fingers to opposing palms with fingers interlocked.

Rotational rubbing of left thumb clasped in right thumb and vice versa. Rotational rubbing, backwards and forwards, with clasped fingers of right hand in left palm and vice versa. Rinse hands with warm water. Dry with a paper towel (without touching the towel dispenser). Use pedal bin to dispose of towel so you don't touch the bin. If you touch the bin, start to wash all over again. Then dispense a blob of hand sanitizing gel onto your clean hands and rub into both hands until dry. Eventually, Phil would wake in the night and realize he had been doing the procedure in his sleep.

Of course, once across the line and inside the ward, the very first thing you do, even though you have not touched any object since the paper towel at the yellow line, is to wash and sanitize in full, a second time. Only then can you touch the incubator, and your baby inside.

Woe betide a visitor who steps casually across the yellow line without following this protocol. It's part of the receptionists' job to remind everyone to wash, wash, wash. Rosemary and Alison are watching day and night. And if they miss anything, a unit mother with the eyes of a hawk – me – would say, 'Hey!' to the transgressor, some uncle who doesn't get what the rules of this place are; some handyman who thinks the laws don't apply to him because he's just popping in to fix a broken strip light. 'You have to clean your hands!' I would growl, furiously.

It was institutionalized obsessive compulsive disorder – but I couldn't reassure myself that it was crazy, because it was real.

My baby was critically ill and vulnerable to the slightest infection. My son might die if someone brought germs into the unit. Death seemed to live in the air I breathed, every moment I was in that place. The handymen would complain – saying they couldn't possibly sanitize their hands every time they walked into a ward; their hands would get so dry they would be red raw. I would scowl and hold up my own hands, scarlet and scaly from washing and sanitizing twenty or thirty times a day, every single time I walked over that yellow line and into my baby's 'nursery'.

And beyond the line? A machine-bleeping world of its own, where the only reality, the only normality, is sick babies.

The morning after I gave birth, my mild fever had vanished, and I felt well. My stomach was almost flat; my breasts had no trace of milk. The fact I'd been pregnant and had a baby seemed unreal. There were only the little photographs I'd been given to prove it, of a baby with a round body – deceptively chubby, I knew; skin and bones puffed out by hydrops, the extra fluid around his lungs and under his scalp. And the memory of the flash I'd caught of blue eyes and brown hair. There was a blank space when I thought about 'my baby'. I didn't know him; I hadn't met him. He was in the same building, just a floor beneath me, but his existence still seemed as theoretical as it had when he was invisible inside me. Still on a high from the birth, I was happy my son had been born in this shiny new hospital building in the heart of London. But I didn't know who he was. And without a baby to feed, I didn't feel like a mother.

Outside, central London kept going. In Egypt, an uprising was happening. Phil and his mother, who'd rushed down from Sunderland, had a dismal breakfast in a hotel across the road. My parents and our sisters made their way into town. Phil brought me clothes, since I had been hospitalized during an outpatient appointment and had nothing to wear.

We were buzzed into the neonatal unit the morning after our baby was born and discovered a world of its own; no, a parallel universe; no, a paradigm shift. A high-level neonatal intensive care unit is one of the most emotionally charged places on earth. That uneasy feeling you get when you go into a hospital even when nothing is actually wrong; the slight sadness when you see a patient hooked up to an IV in the lift? It's that feeling to the power of a hundred.

There was a waiting area which I later appreciated held an extraordinary cross section of every kind of Londoner: ten-strong Hasidic Jewish families praying; oddly vulnerable gangsters covered in tattoos. Many people who find themselves in a neonatal unit have never encountered serious illness head-on in their lives until their pregnancy suddenly goes crazy and the baby arrives sick. Many – like Phil – barely even know what a neonatologist is, or does.

To one side of the waiting room, the nurse accompanying us pointed out the expressing room. Little did I realize that small room was to become a kind of second home.

No one ever explicitly explained that wards here were called nurseries, but somehow we accepted this and it was a comforting euphemism. There are three levels of nursery in a typical British neonatal unit: intensive care; high dependency and special care (in descending order of seriousness). After Phil and I washed our hands and crossed the line, we walked, hearts thudding, down a corridor towards intensive care, Nursery 3, Cot 11, where we were told we'd find our baby.

Thinking about that walk I was to repeat so often over the months that followed still sent chills through me and made me gulp for breath for a year after we were discharged. There was a machine halfway along the corridor which made a sound I will forever associate with the peculiar terror of the walk. The sound was a repeated electronic 'da-da'. It was the sound of a computer monitoring something, somewhere – I never found out what. The closer I came to the sound, the closer I came to my baby, who was behind a closed door in a sealed shell of an incubator.

Opening the door of Nursery 3, I saw a room very unlike any nursery in my imagination. Bright white light, beeping alarms and tropical indoor heat. There were four incubators, one in each corner, two nurses, and a host of monitors by each incubator; one or two other parents in the room sitting beside them. My eyes searched for Cot 11. Everything, it seemed, rested now on this number. I wasn't generally superstitious but couldn't help feeling grateful it wasn't Cot 13. Number 11 was the incubator right in front of me, closest to the door, away from the glazed windows. A young, smiling nurse with dark hair in a pony-tail greeted us. I made myself turn back to the sink by the door, where I washed and sanitized my hands again before I took a closer look.

Inside the clear plastic box I saw not so much a baby as a person. His blue eyes saw me and his gaze had the seriousness and intelligence of an old soul. It was as if this person was trapped in a sick baby's body. He was naked but for a nappy, his hair and his face mostly concealed beneath a colourful woolly hat and ventilator tubing. I wanted to examine every hair on his body but I agonized over whether I should lay my fingers on his incubator, let alone open the portholes to touch this holy creature inside.

There was no crying audible from the incubators in intensive care, just eerie silence. The babies are too premature to cry and, anyway, the ventilators allow no sound to escape and the incubators act as a further muffler. The only signs of discomfort are babies screwing up their eyes, wriggling slightly or fluttering their twig-like legs.

We had decided at Christmas to call our son Joel. Now, a name seemed the least important thing. Standing in the doorway of the intensive care nursery, a young registrar told us that this first forty-eight hours was crucial. If the hydrops didn't go away with diuretics, they might have to insert more chest shunts. I pressed him for more information; what had happened with previous cases of hydrops? 'We don't get them often – I could count them on one hand,' he answered. Trying to sound positive, he said, 'There was a baby who did really well, six months ago.' That, to me, sounded like Joel had a high chance of dying.

We felt so lucky when the hydrops drained away easily (and permanently) with diuretics within days. Maybe that was all, and Joel could now recover fairly easily, like a normal thirty-two-week-old premmie. Maybe he'd even be home in a few weeks. But it wasn't like that.

When Joel was a couple of days old, a nurse took me into the expressing room and warned me: 'The next few months are going to be a rollercoaster. You'll have days so bad you'll want the ground to swallow you up. And then things will get better again. Progress will always be one step forward, two steps back.' In the months that followed, I discovered she wasn't exaggerating. I was grateful to be prepared.

For his first two days Joel was fed intravenously, at first only sugar solution and then TPN, total parenteral nutrition – a carefully calibrated fluid containing all the nutrients and vitamins his body would need. This went in through a 'long line', also known as a central line – an intravenous tube going from veins in the arm or ankle up into the chest, to sit just outside the heart. Until the late 1960s, someone unable to digest food could be sustained for a while with intravenous fluid infusions of glucose, saline and electrolytes, but this was not enough for long-term sustenance and after a few weeks, calorie-starved patients weakened and died. A University of Pennsylvania

Hospital doctor called Stanley Dudrick was appalled by the loss of life and wondered what he could do. He hit on the idea of infusing a solution of concentrated nutrients directly into the superior vena cava, which drains into the heart. Infusions can irritate small veins if delivered through a tiny cannula in the hand – a central line means a bigger vein can be used. First Dudrick experimented with puppies; then adults. TPN was totally successful. Then he was asked to try it on a baby at CHOP.

At two days old, Baby K had been sent for exploratory surgery after persistent vomiting. Surgeons were shocked to find this child had no intestine at all. They did what they could, but couldn't replace her small intestine, so she could not absorb food by mouth. There was no hope of survival. On a glucose drip, the baby girl gradually started to die of starvation over the next few weeks. Her weight dropped to four pounds, her eyes sank in her face, her skin hung loosely and she stopped responding. To trial TPN on a newborn was a highly risky experiment, but there was no other chance for Baby K.

The trial worked. After one and a half months on TPN, her weight almost doubled, and she became an active baby. Dudrick did all he could to overcome every obstacle. When K's skin became dry and flaky, Dudrick realized she needed essential fatty acids. He told her parents to eat a fatty breakfast – sausage, eggs, buttered toast and whole milk. An hour afterwards he took blood from them and isolated the fatty components of the blood, which he then infused into Baby K.

Tragically, he could not keep Baby K alive for long. Aged twenty-two months, she died of organ failure and infection.[1] But her short life proved the efficacy of TPN and so helped many thousands of other sick babies – like Joel – live.

Joel was only stable enough to come out of the incubator for us to hold at the end of his first week for forty minutes, by which time I barely dared touch him, such was his vulnerability. I couldn't imagine what it was like to casually pick up your baby whenever you wanted.

When finally Phil and I got to hold Joel, having changed into blue hospital gowns so he could rest his nappied body on our chests, skin to skin, we desperately beyond desperately hoped this little being would sense that there was more to life than lying in a plastic box covered in tubing, that there was happiness and love.

We were allowed to hold Joel most days after that, increasingly for many hours. The nurses told us he would be comforted by the sounds of our voices. That it didn't matter what we said or sang, just to let him hear us. It was the first time I'd ever sung to anyone who would listen. I unearthed songs from my memory, starting with a croaky, half-whispered 'Twinkle Little Star', tears rolling down my face as I saw Joel turn his blue eyes towards me. It didn't take long to stop caring about someone else hearing my out-of-tune voice. I moved on to 'I Can Sing a Rainbow', then Simon and Garfunkel, and 1980s pop classics. I also read Joel *Winnie-the-Pooh* for hours from the battered brown hardback I'd kept since childhood. My mother talked to Joel daily about what he would do when he got better and left hospital. How she would take him to Cherry Tree Wood, the park near our house, and all the squirrels and flowers and clouds he would see.

Who was Joel? We didn't know, yet. We just knew his gaze remained serious; he still seemed an old soul in a baby's body. Phil and I decorated the inside of his incubator with photos of us so he had our faces to look at – poor thing, he was surrounded by them day and night. We loaded an iPod with nursery rhymes played by a musician friend and left it playing on a tiny speaker in the corner of the incubator. We kept reading and singing to him. Everything is new and different in this world of love and fear – even the nursery rhymes a mother sings to her baby as she holds him in the neonatal unit have to be rewritten. All the king's horses and all the king's men, the nurses smiled, *could* put Humpty together again . . .

We weren't allowed to stay overnight with Joel: there were only a few rooms – for parents of babies who were actually in the process of dying, or who had been transferred from Wales or equally far away. The neonatal unit at UCH is one of a small network across Britain which deal with newborns who need the highest level intensive care. Our local hospital in north London, for instance, had a neonatal intensive care ward, but this only looked after less ill newborns. We lived only a thirty-minute journey by underground from UCH, and every morning we would go in to spend the day with Joel – often our parents or our sisters would join us once the winter flu season was over. In the evening Phil and I would go to my parents' flat for dinner and Dad would then drive us home. Occasionally, I'd get the Tube back to the hospital late at night, perhaps to bring some urgently needed expressed milk for Joel or just to talk to the night nurse. Otherwise we would call whatever ward Joel was on to ask the nurse how he was.

Sometimes Joel had the same nurse for a few day or night shifts in a row; other weeks, there was someone new day after day. We got to know each and every nurse on the roster. They could do anything, those nurses who worked for twelve hours on red alert, with their dexterous gentle hands in blue plastic gloves that had to push feeding tubes up Joel's nose and take blood samples from his heels. They somehow managed to reassure us that Joel was stable and that they believed in him and even loved him, without ever falsely promising that he was going to be all right.

At first I was mystified by the constantly changing numbers on the monitor by Joel's incubator and worried when the numbers seemed to get too high or too low, setting off alarms. Quickly I became mesmerized by the displays and learned what the numbers meant – oxygen saturation in blue, heart rate in green, respiratory rate in yellow, blood pressure in red. You can tell a newbie mother in the NICU from a veteran by how they respond to the monitor. A newbie jumps every time an alarm beeps and calls the nurse; a veteran sits calmly. She can interpret the monitor and, like the nurses, knows not every alarm is cause for alarm. Still, as I was to discover, no one should ever be complacent in the NICU. A stable baby can become an emergency within minutes.

I learned what all the wires on Joel were for: red, amber and green heart stickers performed a constant ECG; a probe stuck to his finger or toe measured his oxygen saturation; the tube down his throat ventilated him; there was a cannula on his hand for medicines; the 'long line', a tube in a vein in his leg, delivered TPN. Before long I was institutionalized, casually talking to nurses about 'desats'. A fleeting desaturation, where Joel's oxygenation dipped for a few seconds, was pretty normal for a premature or ill baby with breathing trouble and wasn't cause for concern. For a long time, Joel was never fully oxygenated, hovering at around 90 per cent saturation. What was a problem was if the desat was prolonged, or dipped further, to 70 or 80 per cent. This, too, was common for an ill premature baby, but it got the doctors' attention when he had a day full of desats – a sign something wasn't right.

Joel's heart rate did odd things, having runs of bradycardia and tachycardia, slow or fast beats, and it tended to beat with an abnormal rhythm. Again, I picked up the neonatal unit lingo and started to notice when Joel went 'a bit tachy'. Yet the doctors and nurses always warned me not to be guided only by the numbers on Joel's monitor. Judith Meek explained that they always judged first and foremost by the baby and his or her clinical signs – how a baby presents in a physical examination. She also reassured us, 'If Plan A doesn't work out, we'll have a Plan B. And then a Plan C. If doctors outline different options, that's a good sign. It's when we only give you one possible course of action that you need to worry.'

Childbirth, however premature, triggers lactation hormones. On day three they started feeding Joel a millilitre of my expressed milk every hour through a tube which the nurses pushed from his mouth into his stomach; an extraordinarily small drop of fluid but a big deal for a sick baby. I wished he could just be fed milk onto his tongue, but premature babies are tube-fed because it's not safe for them to swallow.

Tube-feeding is far from new. As long ago as the 1850s in France, 'gavage', as it's also known, was de rigueur for treating premature and sick babies. Tube-feeding is one of the biggest everyday sources of anguish for the neonatal unit parent. There can't be a parent of a baby who wouldn't shudder at the choking reality of a tube being pushed into their child's stomach through their mouth or nose.

Preterm babies in the 1950s, too weak to suck or swallow, were routinely 'starved' without milk for days after birth, because doctors feared them aspirating – milk 'going down the wrong way', which could lead to pneumonia or choking to death. It was believed the babies had enough fluid, fat and tissue protein to live for substantial lengths of time without food. One doctor remembered a poor baby 'starved' for 111 hours. There is no record of whether that baby survived.[2] Victoria Mary Crosse in the 1950s advocated that a baby's first twenty-four to ninety-six hours should be without fluid of any kind.[3]

The idea of 'starving' babies came to an end when an Oxford paediatrician started to feel increasingly uneasy about it. To much controversy, in 1962, Dr Victoria Smallpeice started feeding small premature-born babies with expressed breast milk soon after birth, using a newly available polyvinyl tube passed from the mouth or nose into the stomach.[4] These days, tube-feeding usually starts as soon as possible – the same day as birth ideally – to help the baby's gut mature. But tube-feeding is not as simple as you might imagine.

Joel tolerated 1 millilitre of milk and went up to 2 milli-litres. We were going upwards on the rollercoaster. But then he stopped 'tolerating' the milk. Before every tube feed of a baby in the neonatal unit, nurses 'aspirate' their feeding tube – drawing up a sample of stomach contents from the tube with a syringe. They then test the pH level of the stomach contents to check it's acidic, as it should be if it comes from the stomach. If it's not acidic, the feeding tube could have moved out of the stomach, even into the lungs. The 'aspirates' the nurses draw up also reveal a lot about the baby's digestive health. If they draw up aspirates four hours after a feed, for example, they'd expect that feed to have been digested – so if milk comes up as an aspirate, something's not right. Now, the nurse found 'bilious aspirates' – a green-tinged aspirate of bile from the gut; a sign that the digestive system is flowing backwards from the gut to the stomach, which could be caused by an infection or a blockage in the digestive system. So Joel had to go back to TPN through the long line.

A day or two later, we came in one morning and as we got to the incubator and asked, 'Has Joel had a good night?' the nurse looked serious and said: 'Joel's bloods show his CRP – a plasma protein in the blood that's a marker for inflammation and infection – is a little high. That could mean his body's trying to fight off some sort of bug. We've had to start him on antibiotics.'

I didn't immediately understand why she looked so concerned. It was only a bug, surely? 'Will antibiotics sort it out in a few days, though?' I asked.

'We hope so,' she replied. 'But we'll keep a close eye on him.' The nurse explained that the problem with long lines was that after being in for a few days, or longer, they could get infected. If a long line infection was suspected, the line had to be taken out, but then the baby needed some other form of nourishment to sustain them, another way of giving antibiotics. Perhaps another long line in a different part of the body. Perhaps we could try feeding Joel milk again, but he might not tolerate that. We were on the rollercoaster, heading down again. A small infection could kill a baby like ours.

We arrived the following morning to be told that a doctor had had to take out the long line at 3 a.m. after Joel had repeatedly desaturated. His temperature had become unstable, too – all this could point to a long line infection. His blood was sampled and found to contain bacteria: staphylococcus aureus. More antibiotics were started, this time into a cannula in his hand. I made myself imagine what had happened . . . my baby lying in his incubator, the nursery lights dimmed for night, then being woken by a harsh light and voices and hands all over his body, holding him down, pushing something through his flesh, not knowing who he was or what life was. Meanwhile I'd been in bed at home, miles away, my alarm set for an hour later, when I'd get up and express milk. The agony of the neonatal unit is the fact a baby cannot fight the hands on them. In their tiny efforts – raising a hand against their face as a nurse pushes a tube further up their nose – is helplessness.

And eventually they get so used to having things stuck into them that they barely notice.

Joel recovered and the long line was replaced, but this pattern of suspected infections recurred time after time during Joel's months in neonatal care. I had to get used to the fact that my baby was being constantly monitored for the slightest infection which could lead to nothing or turn fatal. But even this, and his initial jaundice which required light therapy, were just background to the main crises of Joel's stomach, lungs and heart.

Even with the long line, Joel's aspirates were not normal. They were now often described as 'coffee ground' aspirates – brown with blood clots, a sign of bleeding in the upper gastrointestinal tract, which needed to be taken seriously. An X-ray of his abdomen found his bowel was in strange loops. By the time Joel was two weeks old he was trying nasal gastric feeding again, but the bilious aspirates kept returning. It became obvious that Joel had extreme reflux, which meant the milk fed into him came back up. He could only tolerate very small amounts of milk, tube-fed almost drop by drop. Very gradually, with the help of anti-reflux medication, he started to manage a few millilitres of milk at a time. Feeding by the long line was never far away. A millilitre sounds minute, but as little as 5 ml was a vast challenge for Joel. The problem, of course, was that if he couldn't manage to digest enough milk, how was he going to have enough strength to breathe, to grow? I couldn't understand why my son's digestive system wasn't functioning. I'd never thought before about how fundamental it is to life to be able to digest food. It seemed Joel's body was unable to digest normally. What on earth could we do now?

I'd also never thought before about what an achievement it is just to be able to breathe. Ventilation is not only unpleasant but also risky for premature babies. The membranes in the brain's blood vessels are exceptionally fragile in a tiny baby. The art of ventilation is to maintain normal blood gases – our lungs breathe in oxygen and breathe out carbon dioxide in a constant exchange. If this balance of gases is disturbed, people get ill. If you've ever had a panic attack and hyperventilated, you know how faint you become when you breathe out so much your body is left with a low level of carbon dioxide. In over-ventilated babies, their blood's carbon dioxide level drops, potentially causing injury to the brain's white matter. But if they are under-ventilated, and the carbon dioxide level in the blood gets too high, it can cause a brain haemorrhage. Neonatal doctors try to maintain the minimum possible level of ventilation, but constantly check the carbon dioxide levels in the blood gases.

Under-ventilation had catastrophic results for one family I know. Years after Joel graduated from neonatal care, two grandmothers met on a trip away. My mother got talking to another woman her age, and they discovered they both had daughters who had been through the neonatal mill, and 'special' grandchildren. That was how I met Allie, a clever, sensitive and unpretentious writer with short, boyish brown hair and glasses, her husband Tom, a wiry, tennis-playing researcher, and their sweet twin girls Beth and Emily, born suddenly at twenty-five weeks, just a few weeks before Joel.

With her characteristic honesty and articulacy, Allie told me one evening over drinks in my local pub that pregnancy 'wasn't how people say it should be'. She and Tom had tried to conceive for a long time and had a miscarriage before becoming pregnant with the twins through IVF. They only told friends about their pregnancy after the twenty-week scan: 'I had friends who were calling each other mummy and daddy when they were ten weeks pregnant – we weren't like that.' In Allie's mind, she hadn't really accepted the fact she was pregnant, because she was afraid of miscarrying again: 'I was in denial to protect myself.' Within a few weeks of finally feeling able to enjoy the pregnancy, the babies came. When we spoke six years later, Allie explained: 'I now feel as though I was never pregnant.'

The couple lived in the north of England but Allie's waters broke at eleven one night when she had just gone to bed on a friend's couch in London, where she was staying while she did research for her next book. Taken by ambulance to a high-level neonatal unit, Allie phoned Tom, who rushed to get the first train to London. Allie and Tom found themselves in a delivery room with seven medics waiting at each incubator.

Allie had no idea what being born at twenty-five weeks meant – whether the babies could survive. In her mind, she believed they were going to die. 'I was in a daze. I was possessed; I wasn't my usual self,' she recalled to me. 'My memory of Beth being born is the doctors saying, "Look, look at your daughter," so I looked at my daughter and all I saw was an incubator being wheeled out.' Emily was stuck, and the midwife shouted: 'Allie, you need to push her out now! Now! Now! You need to push!'

Allie didn't know how to push, but she tried. It was 4 a.m. when Emily entered the world. In a flash the medics and the babies were gone; the room emptied, leaving Allie and Tom alone.

A couple of hours after Allie and Tom's twin girls were born, the neonatal consultant on duty came in to tell them they were alive and being ventilated. She did the talk neonatal consultants do so many times, sitting the parents down, drawing graphs, explaining how premature babies' chances of survival and normal development improve if they survive the first forty-eight hours, then the first week. Allie held her open-palmed hands together to show me. Each baby was small enough to fit within them. Theoretically. She wasn't able to hold them for a long time.

Emily already needed the highest level of breathing support. Allie quickly learned what this meant. The doctors were straight about it: this was the last line of defence, they warned, and if Emily didn't pick up soon, she would be in trouble.

But it was Beth who got into trouble first. Within forty-eight hours of the twins' birth, a critical day came for Beth. It was the first of many times a crash alarm went off for one of the girls. An urgently pitched klaxon in a hospital is a signal for all medical staff to run at speed to save a patient whose life is in imminent danger. It's a daily sound in a high-level neonatal unit – the complications of prematurity can occur with shocking suddenness – and parents get used to pinning themselves flat against walls while doctors and nurses sprint from all over the unit down corridors to get to the baby in danger. No one can ever predict what will happen each day.

Later, Allie would get used to the crash alarms, to having to leave her own children, all the team running in through a door as she ran out, giving them space to save her baby from dying. But this was the first time and the most significant. At six that Sunday morning, when Allie and Tom were in their room on the maternity ward, Beth had a massive desaturation. The alarm went off and she was resuscitated.

When Allie and Tom arrived in the ward that morning, the doctor turned around and walked them out of the door to tell them what had happened. Blood vessels had burst in Beth's brain due to under-ventilation: she had suffered a major haemorrhage.

This had created a clot that blocked the flow of central nervous fluid which normally drains out of the brain down the spine. Fluid was building up in Beth's brain and she would need lumbar punctures to try to drain it, then brain surgery at Great Ormond Street when she was just a few weeks old and still far before term.

Allie had no idea of the length of the road she was now going to walk. Looking back six years later, when we met, Allie knew this event changed Beth and the family's lives forever. That haemorrhage caused cerebral palsy and, eventually, severe epilepsy that meant Beth would not be able to walk, speak or eat. But at the time it happened, in shock, Allie felt strangely full of hope. As she understood the situation then, Beth might have some weakness or stiffness on one side of her body. Six years later, Allie reflected to me, 'I was so ignorant. It is extraordinary to me that we didn't realize. There is an incredible capacity for a kind of denial, that things are going to be OK.'

*

Joel was luckier. We were overjoyed when after a week on the ventilator, the doctors thought he could start on CPAP, the less invasive breathing machine consisting of a mask that covers the nose and mouth but doesn't involve a tube in the airways. Finally he was transferred to high dependency, a major step forward. When babies don't need ventilation any more, they come here, on less invasive forms of oxygen and start to establish tube-feeding and breastfeeding. The atmosphere is more relaxed than in intensive care, and the nurses and the parents get to know one another well, chat and hug. It's a place where the hours seem endless, you stick photos of your family near your baby's cot and a mother or father singing to their baby is always in the background. But in a way, many of the babies in high dependency are sicker than the babies in intensive care. Here you find the babies with long-term conditions, sometimes terminal illnesses. And here in high dependency, Joel's progress seemed to get stuck.

Babies hate being on CPAP, but its invention at the dawn of the 1970s was a godsend for the fledgling field of neonatology because ventilating still often had disappointing results. CPAP dramatically cut the death rate of babies with respiratory distress syndrome.[5] It may have helped him breathe, but Joel detested wearing the CPAP mask, and the bigger and stronger he got, the more he fought to pull the mask off. Still, the real trouble started when the doctors tried to dial the CPAP down. You might imagine neonatal doctors go easy on babies. But they push them as much as is safe. From the first day on CPAP, they wanted to see if Joel could manage without it for an hour. The strategy was to try an hour off a day, then two hours off a day, building to a point where Joel would only need CPAP half the time, then a few hours a day, then take it away altogether – then he would graduate to oxygen delivered by small nasal prongs, which would be far more comfortable. This oxygen would gradually be reduced until, around term, Joel shouldn't need any more help and would be 'breathing in air'.

Joel didn't tolerate coming off CPAP well, though. He managed four hours a day without it for a few days, but started to struggle too hard to breathe, so he went back on CPAP around the clock. A chest X-ray showed 'shadowing' which could have been an infection or even a collapsing lung. Having got back to four hours a day without CPAP, at three weeks old he started having too many desaturations and his temperature became unstable; his chest X-rays showed more shadowing.

He had to go back on CPAP continuously. Finally, after a month, he started to wean off CPAP and onto oxygen delivered by tiny plastic prongs attached by tape under his nose for four hours, then eight hours at a time. At two months old, he was off CPAP and breathing in air, but then one day came an episode of respiratory distress and major desaturation and he went back onto oxygen. Because he was still on it at term, he was diagnosed with chronic lung disease of prematurity. This lifelong condition is common in premature babies born at a low weight and often follows on from spending significant time on a ventilator. It wasn't until he was three months old that Joel could breathe in air reliably.

A host of problems ran alongside this. Joel's heart rhythms remained erratic and a scan found evidence of tricuspid regurgitation, a disorder in which the tricuspid valve of the heart doesn't close properly so that blood leaks backwards into the atrium. This seemed to disappear, but the visiting neonatal cardiologist from Great Ormond Street, who came regularly to scan the babies at UCH for heart issues, found a patent foramen ovale (PFO), a small hole in the heart which usually closes after birth but closes late in many premature babies. He said, all being well, it would seal on its own in time.

By Joel's second month, when most premature babies his age were progressing to large amounts of milk through their tubes, and starting breastfeeding, Joel was still in a stop-start pattern of tolerating milk through his tube in small amounts for a few days, followed by severe reflux. Instead of leaving high dependency for special care, the nurseries for the healthiest babies who would soon go home, he stagnated in high dependency. This was when things started to get harder for me. It became increasingly clear that Joel was not doing what was expected of a normal premature baby, or even one who had had hydrops, now resolved. The thirty-two-weeker babies born around the same time as him had now climbed down the ladder from high dependency to special care and started to go home. High dependency seemed as if it was meant to be a transition ward, but week after week went by without any hope of Joel moving to relaxed special care.

At one point, Joel was placed in Cot 13 but by this time, I knew superstition was absurd. As our son moved between wards or things got replaced, nurses would offer me his old identity bracelet or a notice which had been fixed to his cot to take home as keepsakes, and I said I didn't want them. I deliberately tried not to retain memories of what I was living through; I couldn't imagine ever wanting to remember it. So my memories of this time are hazy – less a fluid flow and more a series of near-death and high-pain moments.

By now Phil and I had worked out the doctors' hierarchy. The senior house officers were charming and experienced, the registrars even more so, but it was the consultants who ran this show. Standing out from the blue-pyjamaed nurses, the consultants wore their own clothes. With their practical handbags slung across their bodies as they did their ward rounds (no one else, including patients, was allowed to bring a bag into the wards unless it was in a clear plastic sack, for hygiene), Joel's consultants seemed like intermediaries between this institutional hospital world and the real world just outside. They were able to hold so much, those meticulous doctors. They were the decision-makers, responsible for the lives of twenty babies at a time, dealing daily in extremes of pain, life and death – and speaking levelly and softly to the parents of each child. I hung on their every word and they took the time to talk to us, sometimes for an hour at a time. They found this time to listen and answer me, in huge detail, without ever looking at their watches.

Most of the time in the neonatal unit, I learned, doctors make decisions using complete guesswork. Educated, brilliant guesswork, but guesswork none the less. For example, they can tell you that they think your baby has an infection, but they probably can't tell you for sure if this is the case, or why it's happened, or if and how they'll get better. All doctors make mistakes – it's impossible not to. Considering how difficult it is for a doctor to make a decision in an unclear situation, it was those who decided firmly and confidently, even sometimes with a chuckle and a smile, I liked best. One needs that robust confidence amid so much uncertainty. Neonatal doctors and nurses seemed to me like modern gods, separated from mere mortals by their ability to give life to those who would otherwise die. At times I forgot the consultants were only human and felt a tongue-tied, primal urge to idolize them, to kiss the hospital linoleum they walked on.

As for the nurses, the skill of what they did was almost beyond imagination. I liked the gentle ones, who just loved babies; it was obvious in the way they touched them. And the warm nurses, who managed to communicate news, however disappointing, in a way that wasn't unbearable – with a reassuring twinkle in their eye and never a hint of anything patronizing or officious. Other nurses were superb in a different way: quietly super-efficient; never in your face. Their hands were as deft as a surgeon's and always arranged the rolled towels enclosing Joel in the neatest, tightest of arcs. We knew dozens of nurses by the end of Joel's stay and talked about them at home as if they were friends we'd met at work. We smiled when we talked of our favourites – like Leah, the apple-cheeked, elfin Welsh nurse who always reminded us when we asked why Joel was doing so badly compared to the others: 'Ev-er-y ba-by is an indi-VID-u-AL!'

Little has changed, it seems, since the 1920s, when the pioneering Chicago neonatologist Julius Hess described the
neonatal nurse's role: 'she must be . . . tireless in her efforts to
prevent complications. She must be diplomatic in order to
permit the overcoming of the mother's anxiety, with its conse-
quent effect upon her milk secretion . . . She must be able to
keep a careful record, practice aseptic nursing, avoid accidents
and be cleanly in her personal habits.'⁶

Music can become powerfully associated with emotion. The
innocuous hold music of the hospital's telephone waiting
system will always stay in my mind. You'd probably classify it as
Easy Listening, but the slight charge and urgency in the melody
became, to me, a soundtrack with the mournful, suspense-filled
overtones of a dark psychological thriller. We waited at night,
listening to that music, to hear whether Joel was all right – we
prayed the nurse would pick up sounding upbeat. What frightened us as we sat on our sofa at home before we went to bed,
me hooked up to the breast pump, was not only the occasional
worried voice, but the odd night nurse who sounded distracted
or vague. 'Joel? Yeah, he looks OK,' a voice I didn't recognize
would crackle down the line. These were usually agency nurses
and hadn't met Joel before. There was a total stranger looking
after our child, miles away, and we had to trust them.

Once, and only once, our phone rang in the middle of the
night. Phil, dazed into consciousness, ran for it but didn't pick
up in time. We tried to call back but the NICU line was
engaged. Phil stood quivering, trying the line again and again
for ten minutes. He thought he might have a heart attack. At
last we got through.

'Oh no, sorry to worry you,' the nurse said. 'We just had to
tell you that we've run out of expressed milk and had to feed
Joel some donor milk. It's protocol to inform you.'

One day, Joel projectile vomited explosively, right across the ward. The doctors examined his stomach, trying to work out if it was swollen. They suspected Joel had developed necrotizing enterocolitis or NEC, an infection which is the fear of all who work in neonatal wards. NEC can start suddenly and dramatically, or less obviously with some bradycardia and apnoea. The abdomen distends, and blood and mucus appear in the stools. If it's not treated, lung, neurological and bowel damage can follow – and escalate to aggressive multisystem failure and death. NEC sometimes comes in waves in a neonatal unit, affecting more than one baby at a time. Joel was nil by mouth again, back on a long line. The consultants stopped smiling. I could see how serious this was. He might die.

At some point, during pregnancy, birth, or a baby's first year, most parents of healthy children have to grasp, even in a transient moment of panic, the possibility of death – whether the baby has a brief illness and the parents find themselves rushing to A&E, or the baby's heart rate dips in labour, or the baby falls or chokes or there's a worrying scan. Most of the time, it is just a normal 'scare' and life continues, the child blossoming, the parent feeling older and wiser. But for NICU families, the scares are serious and lasting.

By now, though, I'd been close to my baby dying too many times. I couldn't process the information any more. I didn't go home and research it this time. Joel suddenly seemed, in my eyes that day, a baby in a box, a baby I'd barely held and didn't really know. The doctors and nurses were more attuned to him than I was, I thought. It turned out a week later that if it was NEC, it was gone. But the coffee ground aspirates were back – the reflux was turning out to be a serious problem, a barium study found.

Lactose-free milk didn't help much. One day, Joel aspirated (breathed in) his vomit, a dangerous situation which could cause pneumonia and become life-threatening. After this, instead of a nasal gastric tube from Joel's nose to his stomach, he had to be fed through a tube from his nose into his jejunum – his bowel – in an effort to bypass his turbulent stomach. Specialist nurses managed to direct a tube through multiple bodily twists and turns, through the stomach and into the jejunum – an X-ray confirmed it was in the right spot. The procedure had to be repeated every few days when Joel pulled the tube out. Even on the jejunal feeds, Joel's stomach managed to vomit up clear liquid. The visiting surgeon from Great Ormond Street agreed he needed abdominal surgery; Joel was put on their list.

How sensitive the nurses needed to be to avoid being pushy when it came to empowering parents. When Joel was moved to high dependency, a well-meaning nurse told me I should start changing his nappies and doing all his feeds myself: 'He's *your* baby!' she said. This would probably buck up another mother but it reduced me to tears. Yes, Joel was my baby. Joel was still in an incubator, covered in tubes and wires, and I was too afraid to pick him up on my own. The doctors were still very concerned for him. All I could think about was death. The last thing I needed was to have to pretend he was a normal baby and I was a normal mother and learn to change nappies. I could do that later on, if life was ever normal again, I thought.

I wanted so much for Joel to get out of the incubator stage – he still had to be dressed only in a nappy so that the recession of his chest as he breathed could be constantly monitored. I wanted him to be able to wear a sleepsuit. Finally, he got that coveted open cot and the sign I'd admired on other cots from the start, which read: 'I am wearing my own clothes'. (Some babies were dressed in hospital sleepsuits and if sleepsuits from home went into the hospital laundry, they might never be found again.) When the lid of the incubator is raised and the baby becomes visible, and needs blankets, they somehow seem more 'real'. Although any NICU parent knows this is a deception – the baby in the closed incubator is equally real, just more hidden and mysterious.

I left the ward while nurses put nasogastric tubes up Joel's nostrils and fed them down into his stomach or intestines. It would be almost unbearable to watch him suffer that. But I'd have borne it if I thought it was right. My reason for leaving was that I was afraid that Joel might associate me, his mother, with this torture. When doctors put in a long line, we were always told we had to leave the ward. I couldn't look closely at their wheeled trolleys where they laid out sharp instruments and tubing. I was selfishly relieved to leave but also afraid that if I stayed I'd distract the doctor and make their work likelier to fail. It didn't seem fair to put a doctor under the emotional pressure of having the baby's mother watching. Instead I checked and double-checked that a kind nurse would hold Joel's hand and talk soothingly to him throughout. In the expressing room we mothers discussed what to do in these suddenly everyday moments. Some felt it was best to avoid being there and go in after procedures to comfort the baby, which was what the unit encouraged at the time. Others insisted on holding their babies. There was no right or wrong. It was an impossible situation.

Once, my mother, who visited with us daily, insisted on staying to hold Joel while a young nurse inserted his nasogastric tube, which he'd (understandably, and for the dozenth time) pulled out. Afterwards, my mother was in a cold rage, which is not like her. She told me the inexperienced nurse had struggled, and Joel had resisted. My mother thought she should have stopped trying and told her so. The nurse had kept trying. My mother kept protesting. Eventually, a more experienced nurse was allowed to take over. 'It was right to protest,' my mother still feels today.

Over time, Joel needed so many catheters in his veins that the doctors couldn't stick lines into his arms, legs, hands or feet any more. They were covered in tiny needle wounds. One day, they had to graft a long line into his scalp. When I came back into the room, I asked the nurse how bad it had been for him. 'Well, he didn't like it. He fought a lot,' she admitted, sighing. 'But I talked to him all the way through and tried to calm him.' Numb, I thanked her for her honesty and care.

Joel was deeply asleep, swaddled tightly in his yellow blanket we'd brought from home, his little hands sticking upwards so he could flutter them against his own face, which was turned to one side. He always turned the same way, towards the muted light filtering through the heavily glazed window. It suddenly occurred to me that I could let down one of the sides of his open cot and lie my face next to Joel. It was two and a half months into his time in hospital, that first time I lay my face next to his body.

Phil had taken photographs of Joel, but I hadn't taken one yet. This was so painful that I'd never want to remember any of it, I was sure. But that evening in high dependency with the ward lights low and the babies asleep, I took my first picture of Joel, swaddled, a tube coming out of the top of his head. Then I went to meet my friend Grace for dinner a few streets away. Showing her that picture felt like revealing something too intimate to be seen. But I did, and I laughed and talked brightly, because the reality was too sad to discuss.

I didn't share pictures of Joel looking weak and in pain with anyone else. I left social media altogether for the entire time he was in hospital. I couldn't even write an update saying I'd given birth.

Three months in and no end in sight. Around the time Joel got to term, when he should have been born, he started to make little sounds of pleasure and understanding when we sang to him: 'Aaa . . .'

The NICU was a bit like a strange school, or a prison – new faces would appear from time to time, and then a few days or weeks later they'd vanish, having graduated or been released. Only we and a handful of other parents seemed in for the long haul. Phil and I became thoroughly institutionalized, weary old hands at this neonatal game. Joel was now a kind of mini-celebrity in the unit – all the nurses and doctors knew him and loved him. We told him stories with finger puppets, brought him a musical mobile and hung colourful sheets above his cot, took him out of the cot still attached to his wires and tubes and laid him on a playmat on the floor with some toys; placed him in a bouncy chair on the ward floor so he had some approximation, however pathetic, of normal baby life. On weekends and at Easter the unit seemed to go very quiet and the days felt endless. William and Kate were marrying and the nurses were talking about it, but the outside world no longer existed for me.

One day I asked if I could give Joel a bath. It seemed the most enormous step. He'd never been bathed before, apart from 'topping and tailing' him with cotton wool soaked in warm water. He was so pure and clean, he never smelled. But surely we should start bathing him? The nurse brought in a tub and the particular institutional baby soap approved in the unit. It was safe to peel the heart sensors from Joel's chest for a few minutes and remove the oxygen prongs under his nose (he had by this time escaped CPAP). He had two feeding tubes at the time – one up each nostril, leading to his stomach and his jejunum. We were trying to feed him into his stomach again, but the tube into his jejunum had to stay in because the stomach feeding might well fail and it would be too traumatic for Joel to take a jejunal tube out and in again. These tubes stayed in place for the bath, of course. We held him so carefully in the perfectly heated bath water for a few moments, his eyes huge in his pale face and quizzical, the tubes coiling around him like jellyfish tentacles. It was a success.

But a few hours later, something bad happened while Phil was peacefully holding Joel. It was sudden and unexpected. A nurse sister spotted something alarming about Joel's heart rate and called for help. To me, Joel looked the same as always. But within seconds, doctors were crowding around Joel and all the parents, including us, were told to leave the ward 'Now'.

Phil and I went to a little meeting room to wait for news. We phoned my parents – they were on their way for our family Passover dinner but immediately rushed to the unit instead. As we waited in the room, I ate chocolate. I tried to feel nothing.

A doctor came in looking shell-shocked and told us Joel had a form of heart crisis called supraventricular tachycardia (SVT). His heart rate had started to spiral higher and higher, uncontrollably.

They had given Joel multiple doses of the standard medication but he had failed to respond. Then they'd tried the next best medication but again, the SVT had continued.

Finally a third option had stopped the SVT, a drug called amiodarone. Joel was in intensive care, back in an incubator, and he would have to take amiodarone for the next year or more.

No one knew why the SVT had come out of nowhere, and we never found out for certain, but there was some speculation that the jejunal feeding meant Joel wasn't absorbing nutrients normally and his electrolyte balance was knocked off, which could have triggered heart failure. It wasn't because he'd had a bath, I was reassured.

We went in to see Joel, back in ITU, his clothes stripped off; back in just a nappy. Like a fairy godmother, Judith Meek, who I'd thought wasn't on call that week, magically appeared by my side. 'He's doing well now,' she smiled. It was as if she had waved a magic wand.

*

I returned six years later to the neonatal unit, to shadow the nurses and doctors and try to understand what it's like for them. And for them, it is very different, I found.

Just walking in, the plasticky scent of the handwash and sanitizer turned my stomach. When I mentioned the characteristic smell of the unit to a nurse, she said: 'What smell?' As I stood in intensive care observing, it became clear to me that although I and other patients see NICU staff's work as extraordinary, to them it is, if not ordinary, a matter-of-fact, everyday experience. How could it not be, when you save lives every day? It would be impossible for them to cope emotionally any other way. The whole place, of course, is also deceptively calm much of the time – four silent incubators in each ward; two nurses quietly flushing lines and writing up notes. And yet the atmosphere, as a workplace, is extremely tense.

It was hard for someone like me who sits at a desk all day, drinking coffee, snacking and surfing the internet, to adjust to how hard they work in the neonatal unit. The nurses work for twelve-hour shifts – 8 a.m. to 8 p.m. or 8 p.m. to 8 a.m. – and remain on their feet virtually all day or night. I soon discovered how one's legs ache. Although they are free to go for a break if they need to, they rarely do. During a shift, they hold their bladders to keep toilet visits to a minimum and in the course of those twelve intense hours, they typically take just thirty minutes to wolf down a sandwich and drink a cup of tea, plus one other fifteen-minute break. If things are quiet, they may take another thirty-minute break, but it's often not possible. Not only that, but what they are doing in those twelve hours demands absolute concentration. Constantly. They don't complain; I didn't see a single yawn or a sluggish walk, just nonstop perfect performance. These nurses seemed all but superhuman. After a few days observing at the hospital, I went into an office. Suddenly I saw this office life – my usual working life – in a strange light. This was so clearly a secondary world, a waste of time. What were all these people doing sitting at desks chatting when they could be saving lives?

Of course, observing at the unit was emotional. I only had to look at the consultants to burst into tears when they hugged me on arrival. Judith Meek's email had crashed because her inbox was (as usual) flooded by grateful emails from parents sharing the latest photos of children whom she had treated.

Every time I walked down the corridor or into a nursery, a nurse looked at me with smiling recognition. They didn't just affectionately remember my name and Joel's name, they remembered his diagnoses, his experiences here, and asked again and again to see photos of him on my phone. Judith has such a photographic memory that in one nursery, she pointed out to me the corner where Joel was when he had his SVT. The nurses' faces and names, from all over the world, came back to me, too, and their personalities – the quiet, schoolgirlish ones who kept their heads down and worked immaculately, like machines; the loud jokey ones who made the experience a little breezier; and best of all, the warm and gentle ones who showed my son and me nothing less than love.

I had, for years, mythologized these characters in my mind, and here they all were, exactly the same, as if no time had passed. So many tiny details were the same, down to the little yellow duck-shaped name badge one nurse was still wearing. Now I stepped for the first time into the one room I'd never entered as a NICU mother: the staff room, fuggy with the smell of microwaved food. Judith had to insist the nurses took lunch breaks. We took ten minutes for lunch around a big table, consultants and nurses sitting together (a sandwich for me, a tortilla for Dr Meek), listening to them talk earnestly about what needed to be done that day, that week. Suddenly I wished I wasn't an outsider. I felt awkward coming back not as a patient, but a writer, because my role was no longer typical, and I sensed the nurses felt something was out of place, too. Sometimes it's easier to leave a memory as a myth, to leave the role of patient unchanged.

You need to have a certain personality to work in neonatal care. Not only to be clever and love babies, but because, as one of Joel's doctors, Sian Harding, told me, a neonatologist has to be 'a little obsessive compulsive'. The people who do intensive care work, she said, have all kinds of characters, but the one thing that unites them is attention to detail. Shadowing Judith as she walked around the neonatal unit, I realized that nothing escaped her. She knew which staff were where and what they were doing at all times, even the work experience girl. She knew all the patients, having quizzed them about their professions, their families. And of course she knew each and every baby, examining them with delight at their cuteness.

You also have to be nice to work well with children. Red-haired, earnestly caring Sian Harding was one of my favourite consultants. I always found her a particularly comforting, robust presence. Paediatricians, Dr Harding told me, have been known to call themselves 'the jumper club'. The image of wearing cosy, cuddly jumpers rather than cold, clinical white coats reflects a paediatrician's nurturing nature. 'Being a doctor isn't really a job,' Dr Harding said. 'There's a sense of privilege working in intensive care, feeling you're making a difference to people's lives. When Sian became a mother, at forty-one, it had a profound effect on her understanding of parents' stress in the neonatal unit. 'I used to think, "Why are people getting worried if we have to do a blood test on a baby?" When my son was born it immediately made me understand that extra-ordinary sense of protection we have for our children. How even having a blood test was quite a horrifying thought.'

More than one neonatologist has told me the cases they find hardest are not the babies born with congenital disabil-ities, but the babies who have been healthy throughout pregnancy but who die due to unforeseeable complications in labour. The hardest experiences in Dr Harding's work are the babies who have bad birth asphyxia – oxygen deprivation at birth which can, rarely, happen in an unforeseen obstetric emergency like a placental abruption, the uterus rupturing, cord prolapsing, or a breech baby whose head gets stuck coming out. 'Sometimes when you look after really preterm babies you feel you're defying nature in trying to keep them alive,' she told me as we sat in the consultants' cramped office, grabbing a few moments from the hecticness of her day, 'but when you have a baby with birth asphyxia, who's perfectly formed and been growing in utero for nine months, with the expectation that everything's going to be absolutely fine, and then gets catastrophically damaged in, on occasions, as little as twenty minutes – that, to me, is the worst thing we have to deal with; the greatest tragedy. I feel angry about the loss of all that potential.'

Later that afternoon, as I stood in intensive care observing, the curious tiny bleating sound of an unventilated premature baby rose from within a closed incubator – no louder than a murmur. When I heard this for the first time on my return, I felt alarmed, but the nurse attending explained the baby just needed to poo, and she held its legs up to help, cooing: 'Oh, sweet pea . . .' Changing a nappy with so many tubes on a baby is no easy task, I should add.

Sometimes comforting babies' discomfort is as mundane as that – though at other times, it's not. I watched Giles Kendall – another of my favourite consultants – expertly talking to a newborn baby who needed to be intubated and ventilated because his oxygen saturation wouldn't settle. The baby was in Cot 11, Nursery 3 – exactly the position where Joel was taken and ventilated when he was born. 'We're going to give you some medicine to make you nice and calm – it's all right, just sleep; we're going to do the work,' Giles told the crying baby in a heartbreakingly confident, soothing voice. A cannula in the baby's hand delivered morphine. There were eight doctors and nurses clustered around this baby; they fed the tube down his throat but it slipped out. As they got the tube in a second time, and the baby's arms flailed, Giles continued to hold the baby's head and stroked his arms, speaking sweetly and reassuringly: 'Just relax – it's all right – it's OK.' And he joked lightly: 'Listen, we don't really need your help!'

The next step was for a doctor to feed a central line through the newborn's umbilical stump. The stump contains two arteries and one vein – lines sometimes go in this vein to deliver

TPN and medication, and into an artery to take blood for sampling and monitor blood pressure. A registrar gowned up, a mask over her face and a hair mask. The baby was covered in sterile drapes, exposing just a hole over its abdomen, and given morphine. Having cut across the umbilical cord (which is half the width of my little finger) with a scalpel, the doctor found and opened up the three little tubes by poking into them with a device like a knitting needle. Holding the cord still by clamping it with forceps with one hand, with her other hand she fed a plastic line into the vein with tweezers.

Watching her, I realized how unbearably difficult and painstaking this procedure was – like edging elastic through a tight waistband a millimetre at a time, when the waistband is only a millimetre wide. That is a lot of threading. Every time the doctor thought she had a line in and tried to flush it to check it was clear, the flush got stuck – there seemed to be some obstruction. She stood, sweating, and tried dexterously again and again, for one and a half hours.

Under all the drama surrounding intensive care, I thought, this was the action; the damn hard reality. A doctor working to feed a line into an impossibly thin vein.

Just watching something so irritatingly difficult made me want to gnash my teeth and throw my hands up in frustration. I was floored by the doctor's patience. This doctor told me, 'This baby needs feeds, today. When we know this is a life-saving line, and you know you're almost there . . .' Her son asks her why she's always tired, she added. Her back and legs hurt by the end of each day.

Finally the lines were in and a nurse wrapped a towel around the baby to enclose and comfort him. I could taste exhausted relief in the humid air, but it didn't last long. The father – who had been asked to leave during the procedure – came in and saw a tear on his baby's cheek. He crumpled, asking me if his baby was in pain. I tried in vain to find words of comfort. I told him his child was in the best hands, that the people looking after him were working tirelessly and truly cared. Finally Judith Meek reassured him. A single tear on a relatively healthy baby's face in this place can tear a father apart – and me, too, as an observer – and, I think, the doctors and nurses. The intensity of a neonatal unit is painful to absorb.

Just as important as technical procedures like this is the holistic treatment of babies and their parents: comforting them, getting to know them and treating them as unique people rather than just being guided by the monitors. Nurses in the NICU move babies' hands to their mouths so they can comfort themselves; they also use adult-sized model hands made of beanbags. Nothing can come close to the hold of a real mother, of course. But Judith explained: 'Every moment of being uncomfortable can be counteracted by your mother holding you. The more nurses make babies as they are in the womb, the better they develop.'

The doctors in a NICU also support one another. They're like a family, Sian Harding told me. Rebecca Chilvers, who works at Guy's and St Thomas's Hospital on London's South Bank, is a clinical psychologist specializing in a growing discipline – the emotional ordeal of neonatal care. I wasn't surprised when she told me almost all the mothers and fathers she sees have high rates of acute anxiety. But what did interest me was the fact that a quarter of her patients are not parents, but neonatal unit staff.

What troubles the doctors? I asked her. 'Helplessness,' Chilvers said. 'Despite being real-life superheroes in many ways, it's impossible to be invincible all the time.' It's especially hard for junior doctors, who may not have experienced much death in other specialisms, to work in an environment where there can be many deaths in a week – often highly unpredictable deaths. On top of this, doctors bear the weight of responsibility for the decisions they have to face about what makes a life worth saving – or not. As for the neonatal nurses, their twelve-hour shifts mean they can't escape the raw distress of babies and families. There is so little chance to digest, to regroup. Post-traumatic stress and burnout are common.

Even for the psychologist treating them, it's especially tough. Chilvers has worked before in adult psychiatric in-patients; with people who are traumatized or bereaved. But her neonatal unit job, she told me, is the hardest she has ever done, because she works with bereavement and trauma not after the event but as it happens, barrier-less. The flipside, which she's never seen in any other setting, is her unit's soli-darity: the dedication and loyalty of the staff to one another and to their work – perhaps because it's impossible for them to convey to their family and friends 'what they may see in the course of a day, the joy and the extreme sorrow'.

Among the greatest challenges of her work, Sian Harding told me in a serious voice, is the fact that while most babies cared for in a unit like hers now have good outcomes, some don't. And there are parents 'whose expectations are beyond what is realistic. If you have a very preterm baby who's got multiple problems and is at high risk of having a poor out-come, often people just can't bring themselves to believe that. There are still things we can't do, and one has to understand that.' I thought of cases in the news; how sometimes doctors believe carrying on care is not in the child's best interests but parents disagree.

Sian has mastered the art of talking to parents. If the child might well not survive, 'you have to be professional. The difficult thing is we don't always know they're going to die. Sometimes you withdraw intensive care and the baby may survive in a very badly damaged state. That is very hard. All you can do is offer support.'

And if it comes to death – what then? It's impossible to quantify any death as worse than another, but the worst experience I encountered during Joel's time in the neonatal unit was that of a mother who, like me, held herself tightly together, never saying much to anyone. I thought she was a bit cold, but then I was barely able to smile or talk by this stage either.

I didn't speak much with the other mothers (and fathers) for my first few weeks in the unit. I was too focused on our son. I – wrongly – assumed that everyone else's baby was doing much better than him, because other thirty-two-weekers were going home.

Then, one day in the expressing room, surrounded by mothers talking of their hopes for when their babies would get better and come home, this other mother burst into tears. She shared her story with us.

Her baby had Edwards' syndrome – he had an extra copy of chromosome 18. She spent every day with him in hospital, knowing he would only live a few months. There was no hope of improvement and survival for her son; but also she had to face and live with her grief every day for a long time before he died. I sat with that mother as we expressed our milk side by side and I didn't know what to say.

*

For a long time, no one congratulated my self-possessed psychotherapist friend Eve on having tiny Noah, who survived birth at twenty-three weeks while his twin, Amber, died.

Talking to Eve in the years to come brought back memories for me of how sombrely I used to notice the mothers of healthy babies leaving the hospital weighed down by pink and blue balloons. My friends had sent cards and gifts for Joel but it was ridiculous how much I wanted someone to give me a balloon, to have that 'congratulations' experience. Years later, when a friend gave birth prematurely and I visited her in hospital, I brought her – along with some lavender oil and a sleep mask – an 'It's a boy!' balloon, and saw her smile light up her face.

Noah was ventilated for more than a hundred days, which is a very long time, and associated with a poor prognosis. During this time, he had a brain bleed, and heart surgery when he was just a month old to fix a patent ductus arteriosus (PDA), an opening between the aorta and pulmonary artery which normally closes after birth, but closes late in many pre-term babies. That surgery was one of the hardest times for Eve. She didn't know how they would get to his heart, swathed as he was with a ventilator and tubes. She still hadn't ever held him. But when Noah was transferred by ambulance to another hospital for surgery in a travelling incubator, it was the first time Eve kissed him. After the operation, Noah's incubator was completely covered to block out the light and prevent sensory overload and Eve felt she wasn't supposed to lift up the cover. She felt expected to sit next to the incubator and not look at her son. It was not until two months after his birth that Eve was finally able to hold Noah.

Nonetheless Eve tried to be involved with every aspect of Noah's care – and she felt at home in the neonatal unit, per-haps because she grew up in a medical family: she went to the hospital with her surgeon father on Christmas Day and used to sit sterilizing surgical instruments with his nurse. She knew how to find her way around a hospital, how a ward round works, how the hierarchy of staff is configured. It was not intimidating for Eve.

From the beginning, she had an idea of her son's character. He was feisty – he seemed to want to live. As early as his first few days, Noah started batting away the hands and the needles which constantly came at him. At first, his eyes weren't open, 'but when they did open, oh my God, he used to give these looks that would just kill! He would be looking around knowingly and then he'd fix his gaze on someone, and I don't even know if he could see, but it felt like he could.'

Extraordinarily, despite being in mourning herself, Eve – the kind of strong person others asked for advice and help – even attended a funeral for another NICU baby. A little girl had been in the same bay as Noah and had been doing well, coming out of the incubator, getting her own clothes to wear in an open heated cot. She went for surgery, and never came back. Eve felt she had to go to the funeral. 'It's part of this madness that happened to me,' she later told me. 'I was the only NICU mother who went, and I don't know how I did that.'

But there were moments when she felt weak; perhaps the hardest on Christmas morning. The family had planned to have Christmas lunch at home with Eve's parents and Eve had spent the evening of Christmas Eve preparing it so that in the morning they could visit Noah, go home and eat, and then return to the hospital. 'I guess we were just trying to do something a bit normal,' Eve told me. When she went to bed, the potatoes were peeled and in a pot and the table was laid. At 3 a.m. the phone rang. 'Noah has deteriorated,' a voice said. 'You need to come in – we don't think there's anything else we can do.'

At the hospital Eve and Charlie found Noah on the last resort, the oscillating ventilator. Noah was lying 'like a spread-eagled frog, completely unable to move, his chest going up and down forcefully.' To Eve, he didn't really look alive. A locum registrar was on duty because it was Christmas Eve. He was standing at the end of Noah's bed with his hand on his chin – 'just watching Noah and watching the machine, watching Noah, watching the machine'. He told the parents: 'There's nothing more we can do. This is the last chance. We're just hoping . . . we just have to wait.' They couldn't turn the ventilator up any higher.

At this point Eve's 'positive madness' left her. She was able to take in the gravity of the situation. Every hour the doctor pricked Noah's heel to take some blood to check – sometimes the blood gases would be a little better; sometimes worse.

Christmas Eve turned into Christmas morning and Eve remembers the doctor standing for hour after hour at Noah's bed, only leaving to test the gases and coming straight back again. 'He was like an angel of life,' Eve told me.

Finally Noah turned the corner and started to get better. Coming home on Boxing Day, Eve found the untouched Christmas table, the potatoes still in the pan ready to be boiled. It reminded her of spooky Miss Havisham's halted wedding preparations which become frozen in time in Charles Dickens' *Great Expectations*.

Eve never met the Christmas doctor again but wrote to thank him some time later and sent him a picture of Noah, telling him she would never forget him. She wasn't sure he'd remember Noah, but he wrote back saying of course he did. And that while he had been standing there watching over Noah, he had remembered how Noah in the Bible had lived

500 years and thought, 'This Noah has got to live too.' Letters like Eve's, he added, were what made his job worth it.

*

Phil and I became used to arriving in the morning to find Joel was not where we had left him. Often he had been moved overnight to another nursery for administrative reasons, but there was always a moment of panic that he might have gone back to intensive care or even died. His blood tests showed various abnormalities. His daily problems with breathing and feeding, one infection scare after another, continued to come at us in a blur until we could barely process it all. I heard the doctors telling me from time to time that they were 'giving Joel some blood' but only realized years later that Joel was having blood transfusions. Any one of his problems alone in a healthy child would have been alarming, but with a child like Joel, they seemed to become unremarkable after a few months. By the time Dr Meek told us Joel had a rib fracture caused by metabolic bone disease, a common condition among premature babies in which the mineral content of the bones is inadequate, we barely blinked; it was just one more diagnosis to add to a huge list.

Yet one particular diagnosis was largely responsible for my growing inability to process Joel's ups and downs. It was so major that it made the others pale into insignificance and it changed our family's life.

6

Diagnosis

'I'm so sorry I got it wrong before I knew you.'

HAYLEY GOLENIOWSKA, MOTHER AND DISABILITY CAMPAIGNER

In a paediatric cardiology clinic in Iowa in the late 1950s, a freshly qualified young doctor noticed many of her patients with congenital heart disease looked remarkably similar – like brothers and sisters.

They had widely spaced eyes, sometimes with droopy eyelids; short, sometimes webbed necks; low-set ears; chest deformities; curly hair – and were short in stature. The cardiologist knew of the genetic conditions Down's and Turner's syndrome, and she thought there must be a lot of other genetic syndromes waiting to be discovered. She started collecting data about her patients, writing down on index cards all she could discover about their family histories, their pregnancies, and other symptoms, like undescended testes and delayed puberty. The children tended to share the same cardiac problems: pulmonary stenosis (narrowing of the pulmonary valve from the heart to the lungs), hypertrophic cardiomyopathy (enlargement of the heart muscles), or septal defects (holes between the chambers of the heart). In 1962, at a research meeting in Cincinnati, the doctor reported that she had stumbled across a 'new', previously unrecognized syndrome.[1] Other cardiologists from across America nodded in recognition when they heard the cardinal traits she had pinpointed.[2]

In fact, other doctors had taken an interest in some of these features before. Since the 1880s, patients had been reported in medical literature with webbed necks, short stature, delayed puberty and unusual faces. In the 1930s, Turner's syndrome, which has similar traits, including cardiac abnormalities, was identified[3] – and even after, in the 1950s, Turner's was found to be X-chromosome linked and only affect girls, boys with the same symptoms were, confusingly, described as having 'male Turner syndrome' – despite no genetic basis for male Turner's being found.[4]

The young cardiologist in Iowa had found another explanation. The boys with 'male Turner's' in fact had a completely different genetic condition. And many of the girls thought to have Turner's also in fact had this newly pinpointed condition – which had its own distinctive heart defects and other common traits, from kidney and bleeding disorders to failure to thrive and developmental delay.

The doctor had discovered a pattern linking a group of people – as many as one in 1,000 babies, it has been estimated – who had, until their medical condition was correctly identified, probably assumed they were alone; maybe they noticed that they were different, maybe they struggled at school – but didn't know why.

The doctor's name was Jacqueline Noonan, and the syndrome she identified is forever linked to her, having eventually been given the name Noonan syndrome.

Thanks to Jackie Noonan – today in her early nineties, a sprightly retired professor emerita at the University of Kentucky and still warmly interested in helping people with her eponymous syndrome – Noonan's became clinically diagnosable. That is to say, a doctor could guess that someone probably had the syndrome by physically examining them and taking a verbal history. It was understood early on that this was a dominant genetic condition – that if a person with Noonan's has a child with someone without Noonan's, they have a one in two chance of passing it on. The syndrome also often occurred 'de novo' – happening in a new generation randomly, without being inherited. This was a condition with a broad spectrum: while some cases were obvious and more severe, many people had it so mildly they were unaware of anything unusual about themselves and lived ordinary lives. But it was to take decades, until the latest generation – children born since the millennium – for researchers to find a genetic basis for Noonan syndrome, a way of absolutely confirming the diagnosis using a blood test. And it wasn't just Noonan syndrome. The same process of discovery was happening in the late twentieth and early twenty-first century for a wave of other genetic conditions, too.

Although each genetic condition has its own specific constellation of symptoms, young children who are not developing typically often have strikingly similar difficulties – developmental delays, perhaps a slightly unusual appearance, feeding problems, autistic or sensory processing traits like obsessive interests or craving touch. Today's parents, often desperate for answers, might get a diagnosis of global developmental delay, maybe autism, but instinctively feel there may well be an underlying biological pattern to their child's difficulties. Could their child have a genetic condition which is extremely rare, not yet discovered? They take them for blood testing, enrol them in schemes like the 100,000 Genomes Project in the hope that others with the same genetic profile could be found too, contact charities like Unique, for people with rare genetic conditions, or Swan – a charity for syndromes without names. According to Swan, in the UK each year, 6,000 children are born with a genetic condition so rare it's often impossible to diagnose.[5] When enough people with the same mutation and similar symptoms are found, new genetic conditions get named.

There is, increasingly, another experience, though: a child is given a genetic diagnosis before birth or soon afterwards, because of the explosion of genetic testing now at our fingertips when a scan or some other test throws up the chance of any kind of anomaly.

And this was what happened to us.

It was an ordinary spring day in the high dependency unit when Joel was two months old. Phil had gone to Camden Town Hall to register Joel's birth. Mary, a chatterbox nurse, was on duty and she had got Joel out of the incubator so I could hold him skin to skin. As I was singing to him quietly, a registrar came into the room, and without speaking with me, wrote something in Joel's hospital notes and left. Curious to know what he had written, I asked the nurse to hand me the notes. She read what the doctor had written and her smiley face turned straight. Then she passed me the file.

The doctor had written 'dx PTPN11 confirmed, Regional Genetics Service'.

For a few seconds I was mystified but then it hit me. DX meant diagnosis. This was a genetic result.

The hydrops had gone easily after Joel's birth; all the tests done at the time of the shunt and then at birth – for everything from Edwards' syndrome to cystic fibrosis – had come back 'normal'. Phil and I had assumed that Joel fell into the category of babies who develop hydrops for no known reason. But as soon as I saw PTPN11, I knew what it meant.

I'd first read about PTPN11, the classic genetic mutation found in people with Noonan syndrome, at the end of my first trimester, when Joel's nuchal translucency was unusually large. Back then I'd Googled anxiously for days, learning that this was associated not only with Down's, Edwards' and Patau's – all chromosomal syndromes – but with serious heart conditions – and also another single gene disorder called Noonan's. I didn't know Noonan's was named after the doctor who discovered it – my (false) impression was that it connoted an intellectual foolishness. To me it sounded like 'ninny'. Anyway, Phil and I didn't give Noonan's much thought during my pregnancy or since Joel's birth because scans had found his heart essentially normal – and Noonan syndrome typically involves a major heart defect. Now, this final genetic test result had come back, and it appeared it was positive. My first reaction, though, was disbelief. Perhaps these words in Joel's notes meant something else entirely. I'd probably misunderstood.

Mary rushed to get a consultant. A few moments later, Sian Harding came in and sat facing Joel and me, pushing her red hair off her brow as she gazed into my eyes with concern. 'The result has come back from the lab – Joel does have Noonan syndrome after all,' she told me in a low, compassionate voice, adding a reassurance which comforted me and stayed in my mind: 'If you have to have a genetic disorder, this is one of the better ones to have.' She seemed as surprised as I was by the diagnosis.

Dr Harding showed me a computer print-out about Noonan syndrome and gently took me through the medical terminology page by page, line by line. Facial dysmorphia, including ptosis (drooping eyelids), hypotelorism (wide-spaced eyes), low-set ears, a prominent forehead. A webbed neck. I'd never seen anyone with a webbed neck. Eyesight and hearing problems. A significant chance of congenital heart disease. Abnormal growth, short stature and feeding problems. An unusually shaped chest; possible scoliosis. Kidney abnormalities. Bleeding disorders. Lymphatic disorders (which explained the hydrops). Undescended testicles. Developmental delay, and a good chance of a learning disability. 'I know this sounds overwhelming, but Joel is very unlikely to have all these symptoms,' Dr Harding told me. The clinical geneticist from Great Ormond Street Hospital would come and see Joel, but before then, the first step was to get every test in the book done to rule out heart, kidney and bleeding disorders.

A tiny mistake had been made by chance in our son's genetic make-up. Finally we knew why my pregnancy had been so strange. It seemed unlikely that Phil or I had Noonan's – both of us having been healthy and developmentally normal all our lives – but now I was told it was possible one of us had never known we had it, and had passed it on to our child.

When you're genetically 'normal', you take it for granted. You breathe, digest and grow. My body worked exactly the way everyone expected it to and I hit every developmental milestone without my parents or teachers ever thinking about such things as developmental milestones. I was largely surrounded at school and university and among my family and friends by other genetically typical people.

My parents were 'normal'; they had normal pregnancies. My husband's parents were normal; they had normal pregnancies. For all my character quirks, I was biologically normal and so was Phil. Things like genetic disorders and premature births don't usually happen, so why should they happen to me? – that had been my blithe assumption, going into motherhood. All would probably be normal. And yet none of it had been. My first pregnancy miscarried. My second went crazy. I had learned the lesson that pregnancies are unpredictable, and now I was to learn that so are genetics.

As I was handed that piece of paper which detailed everything that could go wrong in the life of the perfect baby I was holding, I felt myself sweating, and Joel – kangarooed on my bare chest – getting hot too. I placed him back in his incubator and went to the expressing room. There, I called Phil and left a message. I told another mother the news, but that I couldn't believe it. Joel was so beautiful. He didn't look like he was 'disabled'; he had no webbed neck or wide-spaced eyes. I talked to the other mother, as we expressed milk, about how laboratory workers must sometimes make mistakes and how I was going to ask for the tests to be done again. She – a confident mother of a premature girl (which suddenly seemed to me a nice, common medical problem to have) – agreed with me that they had probably made a mistake. I called my parents. They too came from a 'normal' world, of high achievement; they had grown up in a time when children with Down's syndrome were called 'mongols' and often sent away from home. This would be a new life for them, as it was for me. 'He will be even more special, and we'll love him even more,' my scientist father said, his normally matter-of-fact voice wavering. Later another relative said: 'You don't have to tell people he's got this condition. No one needs to know except you and his doctors.' But I knew that wouldn't be possible.

Having been told by the neonatologists that this diagnosis was not a mistake, I accepted it and spent the next couple of days happily cuddling Joel as usual. But then, in the vacuum while we waited to see the Great Ormond Street Hospital geneticist, who was away for a week, I made one of the biggest mistakes of my life. I started Googling. The hospital breast pump balanced on my desk at home, I expressed as I sat at the computer before going to the hospital, looking up Noonan syndrome. Faces flashed up on the screen of people with disfigurements and deformities. They were not the sort of faces I'd ever noticed people having in real life. Where were all these people with Noonan syndrome living? Parents blogged about 'bridges of hope' and 'God's grace' and 'little fighters' and fundraising for medical treatments, and my heart sank. What was so bad that they needed to blog about hope, to build blogs about little warriors, to fundraise? What did they have to fight? I found myself watching their home videos posted online, searching for any sign of freakishness, yet the people in the videos weren't panicking and praying; they were celebrating Christmas and smiling. I couldn't square it, couldn't imagine what sort of lives these families were leading. It all seemed unreal to me, as if these people didn't – couldn't – really exist beyond my computer screen. When I read about terms like fine and gross motor delays, I had no idea what these meant.

On a Facebook 'support group' one of the first posts I read was about a teenager who had Noonan's and autism who had attacked his mother with a kitchen knife. In retrospect, I was very unlucky to come across this post at such an impressionable moment – I have never seen a post like it since – but at the time, knowing next to nothing, I wrongly assumed this was the norm for children with Noonan syndrome. More Googling led me to scientific papers describing children with Noonan syndrome with words like 'stubborn', 'behavioural problems' and 'irritability'. Seek online and ye shall find. And once you know something, you cannot unknow it. Against the pure innocent barely touched being of my unknown baby, harsh words and extreme cases from strangers on the internet became imprinted.

Physical symptoms didn't frighten me. It would be easy, I thought (stupidly), to have a child who had cystic fibrosis, or spina bifida. What frightened me was the idea that my child might not be happy; that he might have behavioural problems and even be instinctively aggressive. I emailed bloggers – strangers around the world – and asked them whether their children with Noonan syndrome were happy. Most (probably bemused by my panicked questions) didn't reply; one American mother answered bleakly, offering no word of reassurance. Another replied: 'My son was fine until he was five, but then he realized how different he was from other children, and that's when the frustration and behavioural problems started.'

Years later I would notice other parents doing this to one another. In a Facebook group, a father posted to express his fears for his sick newborn with Noonan syndrome. Quickly, a mother commented that her child had died.

In inviting the opinions of random total strangers online, I did not for a moment consider that some unhappy people might not be sensitive or might even subconsciously try to bring down others. Suddenly, without intending to, I detached emotionally. For a moment one day, standing looking at the baby with Noonan syndrome in his incubator in the high dependency unit, I wasn't sure I wanted to be a mother any more. In an instant I didn't see the baby he had been before the diagnosis; I couldn't see past the diagnosis. That week, the doctors were worried he had NEC; he was very ill, but I could hardly take that in. I felt afraid, of this syndrome, of my baby, of myself, of the strength of my fears.

There was my pure beautiful son in his incubator and here was a possible future projected onto him: an angry, unmanageable boy. The two were impossible to bring together. The realization came that this bizarre hospital nightmare was not a temporary episode, but the start of a lifelong journey.

It's hard to say whether it's easier to get a genetic diagnosis at the start of a child's life, or to undergo testing for years and maybe never get a diagnosis. Later on, I decided we were lucky, because having a named genetic condition opens doors for all kinds of medical attention and support, which those who have a diagnosis of global developmental delay or even autism, for instance, have to fight for. But at the time, I thought we were unlucky. Had we got a diagnosis for a child, even a baby, whom we had got to know and hold at home, I am sure my response would have been different. But at the time Joel's diagnosis came, I'd barely had the chance to hold him; I'd never been alone or outside with him. I didn't know who he was, we hadn't had a chance to bond, and the diagnosis combined with the physical separation between us made him seem, suddenly, a stranger.

One family came into the high dependency ward for a few days. The parents were full of happiness; they knew their premature child was not seriously ill and would go home within a week. I could not return that mother's smiles – or, indeed, smile at all, to anyone. I stopped speaking to the other mothers on the unit; I wouldn't meet their eyes. We weren't like the other families whose premature babies recovered, I thought; my son was never going to be 'OK'.

Why us? I used to wonder. Why did this weird thing happen to our family, and why with our first-born (which seemed to make it harder, because we had never got to enjoy any normality) when my friends were at home with healthy babies? I asked to see the hospital psychologist, who told me a supposedly reassuring story about a mother she had recently seen whose baby had been born missing a finger.

'You can imagine how hard it's been for her, but the mother is now coming to terms with it really well,' the psychologist smiled at me.

My son had just been diagnosed with a lifelong, de novo genetic disorder. He wasn't 'just' premature or 'just' slightly disfigured.

I found out the name of Britain's top expert on Noonan syndrome (and one of the only experts – I can count on the fingers of one hand, with fingers to spare, the number of British doctors who have a specialism in the syndrome): Michael Patton, Professor of Medical Genetics at St George's Hospital in south London. A distinguished man just retiring from NHS practice, he was among the international group who identified the first known gene for Noonan's, PTPN11, which Joel had. Someone in his office gave me his home phone number; I stood in the corridor of the neonatal unit and called at 9 a.m. one morning. A courteous female voice answered; Patton's wife. 'He's just had breakfast and left the house,' she said, 'but do call back later.' She sounded a little surprised by an unknown patient phoning with a request, yet keen to help. I imagined the Noonan syndrome expert eating boiled eggs in a sunny spring kitchen with his kind wife. How could my surreal distress fit into their lovely life? Later that day, Professor Patton spoke with me at length, and, as gentle as his wife, he told me not to listen to the people online.

I was thirty-two years old and a natural-born worrier; but apart from an episode of depression after taking drugs in my late teens, I had never been seriously anxious or depressed before. You could call me a high-functioning depressive – I'd built a career, had relationships, made close friends. Now, at home, in the long hours expressing milk, with post-partum hormones shifting, and after months of stress, I was separated from Joel and felt myself descending into an abyss of fear. I didn't want to get out of bed any more; my teeth began to chatter all day long and my hands shook in a sequence of panic attacks. 'He's a baby. Don't let him become a bogey-man,' my mother pleaded with me. 'Go in and see him.'

I went into the unit, almost afraid to go near Joel but when I did, I stood holding his frail, warm little body for an hour, my face drenched with tears that seemed never-ending. Joel's only sound was a contented 'Ah, ah'. Other mothers and nurses looked at me with concern but all I could do was cry and hold my baby. Him . . . him . . . him. Everything else went away. Our hearts pulled together like magnets. He knew I was his mother; he accepted me. His love transformed me. Time stopped and Joel and I stepped outside it and felt safe.

Yes, I soon learned, Joel was the only cure. My love for him rebelled against my mind. In fact, I loved Joel with a force I'd never felt before. The more I shrank from mother-hood, the more I needed Joel. Every time I held him, I remembered that Joel was my baby, not a strange mutation. And then I instinctively understood that my fears about him becoming unhappy and violent were ludicrous. I breathed in his intrinsic goodness. I knew without doubt that my baby was the least angry, most loving, sweet, affectionate person I had ever known.[†] But even beyond that, I understood when I held Joel that no matter who Joel would be and whatever he would do in his life, I loved him, infinitely. As I stroked his brow and sang to him in the high dependency ward I didn't know the details of how he would turn out, but I felt the purest trust, not only in him but in myself and in our close-ness, which was so overpowering I knew nothing could divide us. Ever.

† Joel continues to be the most innocent person I've ever known, with an innate horror of anything bad. He is always ready to play and be happy; he never sulks, never bears a single grudge, has never directed so much as a harsh word at me.

Within days, I had embraced having a child with a genetic condition, whatever that would entail. Joel was still the same sweet lovely boy I had always loved so much it hurt. But what was harder was the guilt I then experienced at my initial reaction. It was paralysing and lasted for many weeks.

I thought I was a monster for not accepting the diagnosis easily. My belief that I was the worst mother in the world for having wished my child didn't have this condition was so overpowering that I thought of running away and never seeing my family again. I'd lost my son forever, I believed; even the memory of my negative thoughts had poisoned our pure bond. I was hardly able to speak or force food down. Somehow I carried on. The morning after Joel's SVT, I didn't want to move. Again and again my mother told me, 'Joel needs you.' And again and again I went in to see him.

I now know that depression, anxiety and panic – and a vicious cycle of guilt at this – are classic and understandable responses for any parent discovering their child has a lifelong disability, especially one which may affect their child's brain and development, and especially if the diagnosis comes in a neonatal unit when the parents haven't yet fully bonded with the child. For many, the hardest moments are not necessarily in the thick of fetal or intensive care, but at the point when it becomes clear a child has a disability. When a short hospital crisis suddenly reaches into the long term, the entire family's future changes, it became clear to me years later, after talking to many other parents, with stories like mine, or Caroline's.

*

It was a cold February Sunday in a busy maternity ward when Caroline White, a manager for a beauty product manufacturer, found out her baby had a genetic condition. A blonde, together woman, Caroline had given birth to her first baby the day before. Seb emerged swollen and blue, and wouldn't latch on. He slept and slept, and although no one had mentioned that there was anything different about him, Caroline had 'a nagging gut feeling something wasn't right'.

That Sunday, while Caroline and her husband Simon, also a manager in a business, were sitting quietly with Seb reading congratulation messages, a midwife came to Caroline's bed saying, 'I've got a few concerns.' Caroline and Simon waited two hours for a junior paediatrician. Caroline recalls not taking in the message. 'He said: "There are a few things which could mean Seb has a chromosomal abnormality." I had no idea what that meant.' Later that evening, while Seb slept beside her, Caroline read what the doctor had written in Seb's notes and typed the phrases into Google: 'mild hypotonia', 'flat features'. Instantly Google threw up page after page about Down's syndrome.

Caroline felt disbelief. She had been given a one in 700 chance of her baby having Down's at her antenatal screening but it had seemed unlikely. She had no previous experience of disability apart from memories of growing up near the seaside in Essex, where institutions brought children with Down's syndrome on daytrips. 'I was guilty of assuming everyone with Down's was the same and that there wasn't much more to them,' she later told me. That night Googling in hospital, she felt 'petrified; this was my worst nightmare. I felt sick, my face was hot.' She cried quietly so the other three mothers in the bay wouldn't hear: 'I didn't want to be different.' The woman opposite Caroline looked nice – Caroline shuffled over. 'The minute I looked at her baby I knew Seb had Down's . . . I resented her. She had been given a one in four chance of Down's and I thought: This was meant to happen to her, not me.'

For a few days, Caroline clung to a hope that this wasn't happening. When the consultant delivered the formal diagnosis, Caroline remembers: 'Seb was looking beautiful, asleep in his car seat wrapped up in a white polar bear suit that I'd excitedly bought just weeks before. I couldn't believe it. The paediatrician ended the meeting by handing over some leaflets that made my stomach turn. We had a moment where we laughed but it wasn't funny.' As they walked to the car a passer-by congratulated Caroline on her newborn. She forced a feeble fake smile. When they got home the house was bursting with presents and cards and balloons. 'I hated it,' Caroline told me, 'because it was so perfect, just how I'd pictured having my first baby. Except for one thing.'

The weeks after the diagnosis, there were many bad days. There was an element of pride – they had already announced the birth and now had to 'put on a brave face' and tell everyone this news. She was acutely sensitive to people's reactions; one friend sent a card saying, 'I'm really sorry' – pity was, of course, the last thing Caroline wanted, even though secretly she was feeling something like grief. It was the idea of intellectual disability that was hardest to cope with, for Caroline and her husband. 'It was my first baby; you imagine the future, a tall sporty boy. Suddenly someone took all that away.'

There was the antenatal group to face, with their vaguely competitive emails announcing milestones. There were the Down's syndrome leaflets with inspirational stories of positive journeys – Caroline thought: 'They are better people than me.'

*

In times of need, true characters emerge.

At rock bottom, I discovered, Phil was solid – calm, holding my hand, even able to see the funny side. He always knew Joel would be all right. He didn't Google.

Then there was my mother. As a new mother, one needs one's own mother. When Joel was in hospital, I became a little girl again. I clung to my mother so closely that the salty scent of the soap she used became the smell of my life. I huddled into her on the Tube, holding her hand tight. Day after day, she and my father came to the hospital where they were hailed as the ultimate grandparents, cooked meals, drove Phil and me home afterwards, calmed me with the civilized routine of lives where rooms were kept tidy, phone calls were made and salads got dressed. They gave up their work for those months and together we stepped outside normal life. Mum lay flat on her back on the grass in the park near our house with me one cold spring morning, and we looked at the sky for an hour. Just once, she lay down on the sofa and confessed, 'This is too much for me.' And then she got up and carried on.

And there was my childhood friend Grace, who was there for me – and Phil – in ways I'd never imagined any friend would be. Although, when Joel was first found to be in trouble, I had told her I was 'fine', she had, within days, cut short her career break in India and flown back to London. Now she stocked our fridge with M&S ready meals (we didn't ask her to and she didn't offer – she just brought them). She researched the neonatal unit experience so she could understand it. She called and texted regularly. She came to us in north London on the Tube from her flat in west London again and again, at 8 a.m. She helped me get up, sorted through unopened mail, called people I needed to call (posing as my PA), cooked me soup, calmed me as I cried wretchedly and then came with me to the hospital, where she left me in the waiting room. Most importantly, she had an upbeat robustness, a sense of humour. It sounds odd to say that she laughed at my despair, but that was what helped. She knew me, she was loyal, she was sensible, and she was clearheaded.

I started to adjust to the shock of our diagnosis. Joel was, of course, still Joel, not a list of characteristics on a scary website. I found another mother to email with questions, a talented artist in America who had posted online about having a daughter with Noonan's. This mother responded to an email with intelligence and reassurance. She was a creative, subtle woman – someone who seemed 'real' to me, someone I actually wanted to be friends with, unlike the shadowy random parents I'd been emailing my broken heart to and begging them to fix it. I stopped Googling Noonan syndrome and left all Facebook 'support groups' – making a decision to get all my information from doctors I trusted, instead of the internet.

I started to smile and eat again as it hit me exactly what had been wrong – the unnatural physical separation from my baby. This was the first thing that healed me – the more time I spent holding Joel, I realized, the better I felt.

For a while I pushed myself to the other extreme and started to stay in the high dependency ward later and later at night, until Phil dragged me away at midnight, when the central London streets were empty. It made me feel better to stay, but every time I left, I felt guilty. It seemed impossible, as a new mother in that situation, to find a reasonable balance, to trust my instincts, to know what was right.

The second thing that healed me was the gradual realization – explained to me by friends, family and books – that ambivalence, and then guilt, is a natural and extremely common reaction to the overwhelming experience of becoming a mother. And that's among mothers of healthy babies who come home. For mothers of babies diagnosed with disabilities, and in the neonatal unit, postnatal depression is of course likely to be more intense. But not many people talk about this, and it took me months to understand it and forgive myself, to feel less alone. Some parents don't get sad, but get angry. A fetal medicine specialist once told me how a few parents have shouted and sworn at him when their baby is born with a genetic condition, even launched lawsuits at the hospital. I didn't feel so bad about my own reaction when I heard that.

*

The Great Ormond Street doctor came, a week after the blood test result, to inspect Joel. With great seriousness she took off his sleepsuit and looked at every part of his face and body, then told us that he had no appearance of the syndrome. Although my baby son looked conventionally handsome to me, I was expecting her to tell us that she saw something different, disfigured, about him. In fact she confirmed that he looked 'normal'.[†]

'We are at the dawn of a new era of genetic diagnoses for young children,' she told us. 'Over the decade or two to come, the numbers of families like yours is going to explode.'

The very fact my son had a clinical geneticist struck me as surreal. Having one's child examined for 'dysmorphic features' – even more so. It's hard to escape the connotations of Nazi eugenicists or colonial explorers measuring 'defective' or 'exotic' bodies with callipers.

---

† Which to this day he does, apart from being smaller than his peers.

As a friend whose child had genetic testing once told me, 'That's your blood you're reading about – and it's your child you've given birth to.'

And it does come down to that superficially homogeneous substance – blood – and the hidden strangenesses in it. In a small meeting room in the neonatal unit at UCH, Phil and I obediently rolled up our sleeves and the geneticist almost casually tied tourniquets and drew blood from both of us to send off to a place called the South West Thames Molecular Genetics Diagnostic Laboratory. The objective was to find out if we had Noonan syndrome and had passed it on to our child. Having my blood bottled away that day was one of the most surreal moments of my life. I had spent my life believing I was one thing – but perhaps I was something else.

We spent several weeks wondering if we might have had a genetic condition our whole lives and never realized. But the results for both of us were negative – our son had developed this genetic mutation 'de novo'.

In the story of Noonan syndrome we see the eruption of the age of genetic diagnosis for a new generation. This one syndrome is emblematic of what has happened with hundreds of other rare genetic conditions which have only been diagnosable for a decade or two and which are still barely understood. By the time I started to write this book, when Joel was six, I was like most parents of children with a genetic diagnosis in that I knew my son had a 'mutation' and I knew the name of the gene, but I didn't understand more than that about the biochemistry. I knew Joel's main diagnosis was called PTPN11 and there was also a more specific series of numbers and letters: c.417G>C (p.Glu139Asp). I understood these related to the exact mutation Joel had, within the PTPN11 (there are more than ninety known mutations of PTPN11 at the time of writing, and Joel's is just one of these).[6] I wanted to know what all this really meant.

What was actually going on in my son's body that made him 'different'? In fact, what is a genetic mutation? What did PTPN11 and c.417G>C stand for? I was in ignorance of basic things about my son's genetic make-up, despite being the sort of person who asks a lot of questions of doctors and tries to understand everything.

I started reading the literature and speaking to scientists. My father is a professor of cellular pathology, something I had never even begun to try to grasp. Growing up, the scrap papers I used for colouring and hangman were the backs of printed-out research papers written in an impenetrable scientific language. Now, for the first time in my life, I found the smallest window into my father's work as we sat in his study and he tried to explain cellular communication to me.

Initially, my mind boggled. Trying to make sense of the numbers and letters of my son's diagnosis was by far the most complicated, difficult science I worked through in my research for this book. But eventually, I started to get it.

The vast majority of our human genomes[†] are the same, but there's also space for genetic variations between people – which

---

[†] A genome is the complete set of instructions for making all of a person's roughly 20,000 genes. Each of our cells contains a copy of our genome. In each genome there are twenty-two pairs of chromosomes and two sex chromosomes (XX for females, XY for males). Each chromosome contains lots of genes – individual blueprints for different bodily processes or parts. We inherit one half of each pair of chromosomes from our mother and the other half from our father. Genes are built from a material called DNA, which is made of four simple molecules called base acids. The arrangement of these base acids – our genetic instructions – gets decoded in our cells, and according to these instructions, the body is built and regulated, using building blocks called proteins.

can be perfectly healthy or could cause problems – just like a little variation in the execution of a recipe can make it more piquant, or be disastrous. A tiny mistake in a pathway of communication – for example if a cell dies when it should be growing or vice versa can have huge consequences on how the body works and develops. A response could be triggered by a signal that was never supposed to be sent – like running a relay race without anyone saying 'ready, set, go'.[7] When there is a genetic mutation, the factory of the body is producing an altered recipe on an industrial scale, setting off false chain reactions.

When the PTPN11 gene, for instance, contains an error, the result is that throughout the body's cells in different organs, an important protein called SHP-2 is over-activated. It remains unclear to scientists exactly how this gain of SHP-2 function affects the body, but different organs and areas of development may lose or gain properties; be stimulated or be dampened down – affecting everything from the way cells divide to, it's increasingly understood, learning, memory, cognition and behaviour.[8]

I found out what the PTP, the N and the 11 in PTPN11 mean. As for c.417G>C (p.Glu139Asp), this became clear too. One could fill a book with the details, but suffice it to say that in people like Joel with new (not inherited) mutations in the PTPN11 gene, a single, tiny, randomly accidental substitution in a base acid occurs early on, either a difference in the sperm that fertilizes the egg[9] or in the first cell divisions that create an embryo. The developing embryo starts with just a few cells which copy every time they divide and develop. Anyone who has ever copied out a set of instructions knows how easily a typo can creep in. So, for instance, in Joel's case, a C was written in place of a G. The code is mixed up – and the protein building blocks of the body become different: when Joel was made, instead of glutamic acid, aspartic acid was put in its place. It's a tiny but life-changing typo in the instruction manual which is then copied and copied and copied.

In the case of a syndrome like Noonan's, because the first cells in the body had only just started to be made when the mutation first happened, every body process or part is potentially affected. Many cells in the developing embryo then carry this change – including the 'germ' cells in the baby's eggs or sperm, which could be passed down to the baby's own baby, decades later.

And this problem is all caused by just one minute mistake in the coding.

It hasn't been long that we have had any information at all about PTPN11. It was only in the mid-1990s, with genetic mapping taking off, that the race was on to find the exact genetic mutations which caused Noonan syndrome. Researchers took blood samples from families with clinical diagnoses of the syndrome and isolated DNA for analysis. They looked for a protein which, if mutated, might affect the body consistently with the symptoms of Noonan's – one called SHP-2,[10] which plays an integral part in how the entire body functions, including the heart and overall development, seemed a likely candidate. The gene which coded for this protein on chromosome 12 was called PTPN11.[11] Did the families in the study have this gene? They did. Did other Noonan's families? About half of them did. Scientists had found the commonest genetic cause of Noonan syndrome.

This was just the beginning, though. A few years after the mutations in PTPN11 were found in a large number of people with Noonan syndrome, other mutations were discovered which were less common but also linked to Noonan syndrome. In 2009, a Californian geneticist and paediatrician called Katharine Rauen – a visionary children's doctor at the same university where Michael Harrison had paved the way for fetal surgery a generation earlier – realized that Noonan syndrome was linked to a group of other developmental syndromes – they all involved mutations in one of the body's most critical pathways – called RAS/MAPK.[12]

Rauen named genetic mutations in this pathway rasopathies (meaning disorders of the RAS pathway). Some rasopathies cause other much rarer syndromes which are not Noonan's but are cousins, like neurofibromatosis type 1, Costello syndrome, cardiofaciocutaneous syndrome and the even more obscure 'Noonan syndrome-like disorder with loose anagen hair'. They share common features, from developmental delays to cardiac defects to growth and gastrointestinal difficulties, as well as, in some cases, a higher predisposition to cancer. Researchers are still trying to find new rasopathies (about 30 per cent of people clinically diagnosed with Noonan syndrome do not yet have a genetic diagnosis[13]) and to understand not only why they occur but also why the same genetic mutations affect people in such varying ways and severities, and the mystery of why the RAS pathway commonly affects some parts of the body more than others. A new world of research has opened up, with genomic sequencing now easily done by a machine within a day, compared to the years of painstaking manual checking needed at the turn of the twenty-first century, and databases which automatically filter out potential disease-linked mutations from those which don't cause problems. Previously unknown mutations are being identified year on year.

The point is that this tale of the discovery of the genes for my son's particular condition is emblematic of the genetics revolution over the last few decades. We now have more and more children growing up with newly identified, often very rare, genetic mutations. Advances in testing for Noonan's happened not in isolation but with the completion of the Human Genome Project in 2003 in which researchers around the world spent thirteen years sequencing the whole human genome for the first time, and the 100,000 Genomes Project which has sequenced the genomes of people with rare diseases and their families, searching through haystacks for common needles.

So I started to understand, at last, something of the science, and the modern history of genetic discovery which has so powerfully changed my family's life. But there's another thing I didn't understand when I got the diagnosis and still don't understand. I'm not alone in this. Consultant geneticist Professor Lucy Raymond, from the University of Cambridge, told me the commonest question families ask her when they get such a diagnosis is: 'But what does this *mean*?' Her practice is changing, Professor Raymond explained to me. In the past, doctors' mission was trying to identify the gene that had caused a child's mystery disorder. Today, geneticists have often found the variant, but need to counsel families asking the deeper question: 'So what?'

It's easy for a doctor to give a child a label, but hard for anyone to predict how a genetic condition will affect someone. When Joel was five and I was ready, I rejoined the Noonan syndrome Facebook groups and found many answers to my questions – as well as enormous positivity. Before the world got online in the late 1990s, it was hard for families to find any information about little-understood syndromes like Noonan's. A couple of decades later, as I discovered at the start of my journey, you can find anything you search for on the internet, much of it totally misleading. Happily, though, there are now thousands of people all over the world who share useful information in the main Noonan syndrome Facebook groups and they grow exponentially, day by day.

Families tend to know more about rare genetic conditions than general practitioners and even many specialists. Phil and I soon got used to hospital doctors looking up our child's syndrome on Wikipedia. Many people with Noonan's have debilitating pains in their legs and gut problems – but at the time of writing, doctors seem to know virtually nothing about this.

The pace of discovery is so dizzying that one consultant geneticist at a children's hospital cheerfully told me it's a struggle to keep up with her own field. Again, to use Noonan's as an example of one of so many syndromes: in the last few years, as more mutations associated with Noonan's have been discovered, and more children have undergone genetic testing, and more people are pooling knowledge on social media, the number of children being diagnosed with Noonan's in economically developed countries has soared (Noonan's Facebook support groups in English are overwhelmingly North American). And in many cases, their mother or father has then found out they also have the same condition, one they had never heard of before. One great-grandmother in America – 4 feet 11 inches tall, with a characteristic facial appearance and various health issues – finally got a clinical diagnosis at the age of eighty-nine in 2017, when she saw a cardiologist who connected her symptoms with those of her daughter, granddaughter and great-granddaughter with Noonan syndrome.

Another story I love is that of the charming Dutch scientist Judith Van de Meerakker. As an infant, Judith was diagnosed with congenital heart defects and she had had three open heart surgeries by the age of three. It was her own personal experience as a heart patient that led her, in adulthood, to decide to study for a PhD in the genetics of congenital heart defects. During her research, Judith read about Noonan syndrome. It sounded like something that could potentially apply to her – not only did she have heart defects, but she had always known she was 'somehow different'. Of course, those who research medical problems easily worry that they have the symptoms of dozens of rare disorders. Judith's colleague, though, agreed that she really might have Noonan's. So at the age of thirty-one, she got herself a blood test. It turned out she had a mutation in PTPN11. After the diagnosis, various traits – low-set ears, bruising quickly, late puberty, lymphatic problems, ADHD and cognitive difficulties – fell into place like pieces of a jigsaw puzzle.

In the 1950s and 1960s, it was considered quite normal to send a disabled child to an institution. A 1956 edition of a standard medical textbook, *Sick Children*, by Great Ormond Street Hospital physician Donald Paterson, discusses the parenting of 'the feeble-minded and imbeciles', not to mention 'the idiot'. (Obviously, none of these are categories any child in Britain would be described under today. But in the early twentieth century, these were not intended as insults but as specific psychiatric terms. An 'idiot' was a person with an IQ of 0–25 and an 'imbecile' had an IQ of 26–50, while a 'moron' IQ was 51–70.) The doctor wrote: 'Idiots and many imbeciles are best cared for in institutions, especially if there are other children at home who may be neglected because of the demands made by the defective.' Children with Down's syndrome, described as 'mongols', he wrote, 'cannot be trusted to any great extent and do not prove useful members of society'.[14] My mother had a friend, in the 1970s, who with her husband chose to send their newborn with Down's syndrome to be fostered from birth. Later, when my mother asked her how her son was, the friend replied: 'What son?'

It's hard to imagine today – but then I found out that disabled children have been 'put away' in my lifetime too.[15] The harrowing documentary *The Silent Minority*, broadcast on British TV in 1981, revealed that in Britain, disabled children – the blind, the deaf, those with cerebral palsy (then called 'spastics'), those with learning disabilities and those with genetic conditions including, very likely, Noonan syndrome – might well live their lives drugged in barren wards. One little boy in the film, considered troubled but just desperate for attention, was tied standing to a post for five hours a day. Blind children clung together for comfort. These unspeakably neglected, 'sub-normal' children turned into despairing adolescents who sat all day rocking and chewing their clothes, sometimes in solitary confinement. By adulthood, the men were lined up in wheelchairs naked, covered only by sheets, for rows of baths, and slept in vast dormitories.

In the children in the film, I saw the bright eyes and awkward movements of my own son – and I saw how a boy like him could have ended up in a different time, with different parents who abandoned him to a place almost too hellish to be believed. After I watched the film I felt haunted by the helpless boy tied to the post in an empty ward. Where is he now?

That era has waned, replaced by buzzwords like 'inclusiveness' and 'diversity'. Modern doctors who treat children with disabilities have to try to be inoffensive, right down to the language they use – for example, where do you draw the line in calling someone 'normal'? 'In science and medicine we do say "normal" and "abnormal" but it's actually not terribly helpful, and we've got to be very careful not to in any sense be derogatory,' Professor Raymond told me. We were speaking on the phone, and she confessed this was particularly difficult because she couldn't be guided by my facial expressions; I gleaned that it was hard for her to know if her language about difference was respectful enough. It must be hard for a doctor, I replied sympathetically. As a mother, I have always sensed others' fear of saying the wrong thing when speaking about my child with a genetic condition, and felt sorry for them. Parents like me could so easily take offence; others tiptoe around us.

The truth is that the notion of a genetically different child as an aberration is still often there in the background, however masked by patronizing political correctness and however unconscious. Once, a doctor examining Joel called for her student to observe, and remarked on his distinctive facial features, which I thought barely noticeable (and more objectively, judging from strangers on the street, nobody has ever stopped to look twice at him and ask if there is something wrong with him). If you're scrutinizing anyone's face, you could find abnormalities, surely? Or take the holiday club leader who, on hearing I had a child with a disability, quickly started talking about why they couldn't cater for such a child easily; he said he would call back, then never did.

*

We suddenly know facts about ourselves and our children that previous generations didn't know. And yet beyond the basic numbers and letters of a gene's location and some common symptoms, we still know almost nothing. The consultant geneticist Lucy Raymond told me that some parents of children with developmental delays don't want to have the child genetically tested – they would rather not know the answer. But now that we're often linking developmental problems with genetic conditions which may – like Noonan's – have a high chance of cardiac or other life-threatening problems, the decision to remain in ignorance could arguably become a form of child neglect. On the other hand, sometimes we know more than we can understand. Exactly how genetic disorders affect the brain, in particular, is still a mystery. We are not defined by our genetic blueprints; nurture plays a major role in shaping a person, too. It's tempting, when your child has a genetic condition, to think every trait or behaviour comes down to that. But where does a syndrome end and a person begin? And who's to say which of our 'abnormal' genes is a problem, and which is an evolutionary step forward from the homogeneous masses?

There are large but unknowable numbers of people who have genetic anomalies and have no idea, because the effects are so mild – or even non-existent – in their case. So how much do we want to know, and where should we draw the line in labelling someone as having a 'disorder', given that we all have genetic variations, and it's often not clear which mutations are medically significant?

Genetic diagnosis before birth, given all this, is a strange form of knowledge.

When I revisited the fetal medicine unit at UCH as a journalist, I observed two women having chorionic villus sampling (CVS) in early pregnancy, an invasive procedure to test for chromosomal abnormalities in which a needle is inserted through the abdomen to get a sample of cells from the placenta (amniocentesis, the other type of invasive test, takes a sample from the amniotic fluid). The needles were as long as rulers; the women lay facing the wall so they could not see them, while the husbands looked on, visibly aghast. The first woman was almost silent throughout, her only sign of emotion covering her eyes when a few tears crept out. The registrar who did the procedure told me he didn't get butterflies, though 'there's a lot of consequence on the end of that needle'.

A private blood test had found the second couple's fourteen-week baby almost certainly had Down's syndrome. The mother had previously had a CVS which found no genetic condition and then miscarried – 'poor thing', the midwife Georgina said before they came in. Now, the mother asked for the ultrasound screen set up for patients to be turned off. 'I don't want to see the baby,' she said. Her husband held her hands and stroked her face; she cried quietly. After they thanked Professor Peebles and went to recovery, Georgina came back in to say the mother was upset – she wanted a vacuum aspiration (in which the pregnancy is suctioned out via the cervix) but she was nearing the hospital's time limit for this procedure, after which she would have to go under anaesthetic and have the fetus pulled out using forceps, or take medicine to stimulate contractions and deliver through the vagina – effectively, labour.

The history of searching for genetic conditions in unborn babies is a very new one, and inextricably linked with abortion politics. The development of screening and diagnosis for one genetic syndrome, above all, is the thread through which we can trace this history. Down's syndrome is the commonest and highest-profile disability diagnosed before birth. It has always been the main target of antenatal screening programmes, arguably not for any good reason – it's far from the most serious condition which could affect a child, but it's a common one we've worked out how to spot quite easily in utero.

Down's syndrome's genetic basis, an extra copy of the twenty-first chromosome, was only identified in 1959. Although nineteenth-century scientists discovered chromosomes when looking at cells under the microscope,[16] it wasn't until the 1950s that the twenty-three pairs of the human chromosome were mapped for the first time. But a century earlier, a distinct group of people with characteristics including 'idiocy', flat, broad faces, 'thick and indistinct' speech, feeble circulation and 'a lively sense of the ridiculous' was first described by Dr John Langdon Down in 1862, and although he called them 'mongols', his name was, by the 1960s, attached to the syndrome.[17]

Once scientists had identified the forty-six normal human chromosomes, genetic testing became a reality. In 1956, fetal cells from amniotic fluid were analysed to predict a baby's sex for the first time – XX for a girl versus XY for a boy.[18] In 1961, a chromosomal abnormality – triploidy, a very rare condition in which there are three instead of the usual two sets of each chromosome – was found for the first time in an aborted fetus.[19] Then, in spring 1966, American scientists studying the genetics of mental retardation took a tiny amount of amniotic fluid from a pregnant woman. Having grown the fetal cells in a Petri dish, they stained the chromosomes different colours to differentiate them, and analysed them under a microscope, aiming to identify a genetic disorder.[20] The first prenatal diagnosis of Down's syndrome soon followed, followed by other genetic conditions.

The first known abortion after a genetic test is recorded in a 1968 case report from a Brooklyn medical centre linked to the University of New York. We know next to nothing about the twenty-nine-year-old pregnant woman, apart from the bare facts of the medical history. Six years before, she had miscarried a girl whose features indicated she had Down's syndrome. A healthy child was born in 1963. Two years later, her next child, a boy, was born and diagnosed with Down's syndrome. With multiple holes in the heart, he died in hospital after an attempt at surgery, aged just five months old. Now the woman was pregnant again, and she asked for prenatal testing. As she approached her third trimester, an amniocentesis discovered she was carrying a boy, with Down's syndrome. In the last few days that a termination was allowed, she ended the pregnancy. Nothing more is known, other than that she wanted to try again for a baby, with genetic testing again next time.[21]

Some chromosome abnormalities, like trisomies 13, 18 and 21 (Patau's, Edwards' and Down's syndromes), involve three (tri) copies of a chromosome instead of two. Others are sex-chromosome mutations, like Turner's and Klinefelter's. And in other cases called translocations, there's the right number of chromosomes, but they are rearranged. Smaller chromosomal changes are known as microdeletions or microduplications.[22] And then there are 'single gene' disorders like the rasopathies, cystic fibrosis, or fragile X, in which one tiny genetic mutation can cause major changes. The need to get a sample from the fetus to test for genetic anomalies saw amniocentesis and CVS develop into a routine part of antenatal practice through the 1970s and 1980s.[23]

At the same time as taking samples of fetal tissue for pre-natal diagnosis was becoming common, the idea of a blood test for fetal abnormality developed as biochemical 'markers' for genetic conditions in the fetus were identified in maternal blood. In 1972, the same year that Stuart Campbell made the first ultrasound diagnosis of a disorder, others discovered that a protein made by the developing fetus, called alpha-fetoprotein (AFP), was raised in amniotic fluid in cases of anencephaly and spina bifida, both open neural tube defects. Soon AFP was detectable in mothers' blood, too.[24] In 1975, Campbell diagnosed the first case of spina bifida using ultra-sound, and the idea of antenatal screening using a combination of testing the mother's blood for unusual AFP levels, scanning and amniocentesis emerged, first for open neural tube defects and then, in the 1980s, for Down's syndrome, in which AFP levels (and other markers) are often different in the mother's blood.[25] Prenatal diagnosis led to soaring numbers of terminations of babies with open neural tube defects and Down's syndrome.[26]

The next major move which made it even easier to flag up Down's syndrome in utero came about by coincidence. In 1991, a patient came to Kypros Nicolaides with a tragic history. She had lost baby after baby to rhesus disease – her blood was rhesus negative, destroying her babies' rhesus positive blood. Nicolaides decided to try a bone marrow transplantation at only twelve weeks' gestation – taking bone marrow from the mother and giving it to the fetus, in an attempt to change the baby's blood group. As he carefully scanned the baby, Nicolaides noticed it had a lot of fluid behind its neck. This wasn't an expected complication of rhesus disease so early in pregnancy.

Anxious to help the mother, Nicolaides went ahead with the transplant, but also removed a sample of amniotic fluid for chromosomal testing. This revealed the baby had an extra chromosome – a diagnosis of Down's syndrome. The thought struck the doctor: 'Could it be that this large collection of fluid behind the neck actually is a marker for Down's?' The mother aborted the fetus with Down's syndrome. She went on to get pregnant again and, due to her rhesus negative blood, Nicolaides started blood transfusions in the first trimester. The baby survived and grew up to become a ballet dancer.[27]

By chance, Nicolaides had stumbled across a common marker for Down's syndrome, cardiac problems – and Noonan syndrome. He wasn't, in fact, the first to make the connection, but he was the doctor who made the idea take off.[28] By the millennium, the twelve-week nuchal translucency scan measuring the collection of fluid under the baby's neck was a routine part of antenatal screening around the world.

But during the early 2000s, a far more accurate way of finding Down's – and other genetic conditions – was gaining pace. This game-changer for prenatal diagnosis was a total evolution of the maternal blood tests developed in the 1970s and 1980s. The seed for it started back in the 1890s, when a German pathologist, Georg Schmorl, was performing autopsies of seventeen women who had died from pre-eclampsia and found strange cells in their lungs.

Schmorl realized that these cells came from the placenta – increased 'fetomaternal trafficking' is linked to eclampsia. It was also proof that fetal cells pass into the mother's body. Today we know that about one in every million cells in the mother's circulation comes from the fetus. A hundred years after Schmorl's discovery, scientists figured out how to measure fetal DNA in the mother's blood – today this new, non-invasive prenatal testing (NIPT) for genetic disorders is rolling out around the world.[29] A simple blood test available from ten weeks of pregnancy, it has a 98 per cent plus accuracy rate for detecting trisomy 21.

With genetic and ultrasound advances, we are now making diagnoses in utero earlier and more easily than ever before. And on the horizon as I write is a new era which will revolutionize prenatal screening and diagnosis and introduce even more ethical conundrums: gene editing for congenital conditions. In the not too distant future, parents may well not only get their fetus's whole genome sequenced in utero,[30] but if a disorder is found they may have the option to get the child's DNA 'fixed' before birth – or not.

I learned first-hand that a child with a syndrome is a joy, like any child. And when Joel was a toddler, at a support group for children with disabilities and their parents, I got to know several families whose children had Down's. As they told me their stories of diagnosis – while my adorable son played with their adorable children – these parents told me they were deeply offended by the way society screens unborn babies for genetic differences. The very naming of tests for Down's – Tranquillity, Harmony – and the routine leaflets' language about the 'risk' of Down's give a clear message to prospective parents (which once frightened me, too): babies with genetic anomalies are undesirable.

Down's syndrome termination rates are a useful prism through which we can see our society's attitude to congenital disability. In England in 2014, an estimated 90 per cent of babies diagnosed prenatally with Down's were aborted.[31] Famously, in Iceland virtually 100 per cent of babies identified with Down's in utero are now aborted.[32] (Of course, some parents who would not terminate refuse testing.)

Late terminations on medical grounds are an emotive issue. In Britain, with extremely premature babies savable by the early 1990s, the UK Abortion Act of 1992 brought the gestational age for non-medical terminations down from twenty-eight to twenty-four weeks. Abortion after twenty-four weeks on medical grounds has been permitted since 1992 for a child with a risk of being 'seriously handicapped' due to 'physical or mental abnormalities', as well as for a pregnancy where the mother's physical or mental health is at risk. This means termination for medical reasons can happen, at a doctor's discretion, right up to term. The procedure is the same as for earlier abortions. Labour is stimulated or the pregnancy is removed using forceps under general anaesthetic, but after twenty-two weeks, the fetus's heart is stopped by injection at the start or during the procedure, so that it is not born alive.

What legally constitutes a 'serious handicap' is not defined,[†] so babies with Down's, which some argue is not a severe disability, are being aborted after twenty-four weeks – twenty-one of them in 2016.[33] A child with Noonan's syndrome could also be aborted right up till forty weeks' gestation in Britain.

Society's understanding of where life begins has changed, and along with it, ideas about abortion have been challenged. The ultrasound pioneer Stuart Campbell spoke to me of 'this invidious situation where at one end of a corridor you have a neonatologist in an intensive care unit, trying to keep a twenty-four-week-old alive and the other end of the corridor you have people terminating a twenty-four-week-old. That is illogical and stupid.'

Campbell is pro-choice, but he has campaigned to reduce the UK's time limit for terminations for non-medical reasons from twenty-four to eighteen weeks and would like to see it reduced to twelve weeks ideally. The more 'real' the fetus has become thanks to fetal medicine, the more attention society has paid it. Campbell's work observing babies in utero changed his perspective. 'I didn't feel so strongly until I started seeing fetuses at twenty to twenty-four weeks; the complexity of the behaviour,' he told me.

To face giving one's unborn baby, by the time they are kicking, an injection starkly described by the British Pregnancy

† Terminations on medical grounds for very minor disabilities are vanishingly rare in Britain but do happen: in 2016 there were nine recorded for the 'principal medical condition' of cleft lip/palate. (https://www.gov.uk/government/uploads/system/uploads/attachment_data/file/652083/Abortion_stats_England_Wales_2016.pdf, accessed 31 January 2018).

Advisory Service's online patient information as 'feticide',[34] is a desperately hard situation to consider and undergo. A late termination is a heartbreaking choice which deserves the utmost compassion. And making the decision to end a pregnancy diagnosed midway with serious problems is, due to fetal medicine's new powers to diagnose, a situation many parents find themselves in; it's just hardly ever discussed in public.

Ultimately, it's difficult to make a decision without knowing the 'truth' of a condition – and although in some cases a baby will have no chance of surviving far beyond birth or any quality of life, the truth of many genetic syndromes is immensely variable. Down's syndrome is, again, a useful example to delve into because (like so many genetic syndromes, including Noonan's) what people 'know' about it is so different. At one end of the scale, Down's families and disability rights groups say a life with Down's is absolutely worth living. As scientific possibilities for catching Down's before birth evolved, Down's awareness did, too. Being able to diagnose and, sometimes, treat babies found to have disabilities before birth has coincided with the rise of disability rights. What we still call 'abnormalities' or 'anomalies' in the fetus are what we speak of more sensitively after birth as 'disabilities' and 'diversity'.

A 1979 book, *Prevention of Handicap and the Health of Women*, expressed with concern how children with Down's were living for longer, and that if the new science of amniocentesis could prevent the births of even 10 per cent of babies with Down's, it 'would be a contribution to a very grievous problem'.[35] But we are learning more about 'abnormality' and its gifts. A person with Down's born in a developed country in the twenty-first century has heart surgery if needed and can typically expect to live into their fifties, perhaps their seventies. Given the opportunity, some live independently of their families, with a degree of support; they have careers, relationships and busy social lives.[36]

In 2015, a petite blonde woman in her forties stood in front of a TEDx audience and declared passionately: 'The doctor predicted that I would be lucky to be able to tie my own shoes or write my own name.' Karen Gaffney, from Oregon, has a science degree, an honorary doctorate and is a champion swimmer who has crossed the English Channel in a team relay event. She also has Down's syndrome, and in her speech she explained why she was wary of the race to 'find newer, faster ways to test for Down's syndrome before birth'. Gaffney articulately described how families and grassroots campaigners have, over the past forty years, 'opened the doors' for a new generation of people with Down's to have an education and become valued citizens. (There's still far to go. Viral videos celebrating people with Down's syndrome's achievements are heartwarming, but a disabled child who does not do 'normal' things is no less deserving of a life.)

Caroline White, who struggled when her son Seb was born with Down's, is a forthright blogger on disability today. She is not afraid to say: 'Had I been told when I was pregnant, I would have trusted the people in the white coats and terminated; that's what people do. Now I can't believe I'd have thought that.' Caroline told me she perceived a 'sad irony' in so many terminations for Down's while inclusion in schools and society grows. 'Seb's friends don't even know he has Down's. If you asked them to describe him they would say: sporty, funny, polite. I'm pro-choice but it needs to be pro-informed choice. People need to be aware of what it means to have Down's in the twenty-first century.'

Jane Fisher, director of the Antenatal Results and Choices (ARC) charity, which counsels pregnant women when a fetal anomaly is detected, supports women's right to terminate babies with Down's after twenty-four weeks and strongly disagrees that women are influenced to terminate. 'This may be controversial, but Down's syndrome isn't an insignificant condition,' she told me. 'There's sometimes a tendency from those who have children with Down's syndrome to believe that women are making ill-informed decisions when they choose to end the pregnancy, that they're pushed into it based on out-of-date information, or that they're making a selfish decision because they want the perfect baby, that they're not prepared to put the extra work in – and we would categorically counter that.'

An article in *The Cut* by journalist Jen Gann tells of how, when she became pregnant, she and her husband had genetic testing to see if they were carriers for cystic fibrosis, a condition in which the body mishandles sodium and chloride, leading to mucus-filled lungs and other organs – a very tough life in and out of hospital. In 2016, half of the reported deaths for cystic fibrosis were in people under thirty. No one called to tell Gann and her husband the result, that they were both carriers. It was only after their son was born and found to have cystic fibrosis that the clinic's mistake came to light. In the article, Gann wrote of her love for her son, and of how if she had known he had this condition, she would have ended the pregnancy.

She wrote: 'Parents like me often feel betrayed by their child's cystic fibrosis diagnosis. Maybe there was medical malpractice, maybe an inherited mutation so rare it wasn't detected prenatally. Other parents have chosen to avoid any kind of testing, believing it's their destiny to embrace whatever God or fate or genetics deals them. I'm horrified by the sanctimony that often accompanies this acceptance, especially when it's admired, especially when it's offered up by mothers who don't "believe" in prenatal testing or who have more than one child with cystic fibrosis. The women who willingly made choices that were never presented to me and chose a child's suffering. Sometimes I hate them.'

She continued: ' "I love my child just the way he is," is a sentiment often put forth, fiercely, by the parents of sick or disabled kids. It's not hard to understand the intention – every parent wants to make it clear that no challenge renders their love conditional. But given the choice, if one existed, I would have Dudley another way: healthy.' [37]

I admired the honesty of Jen Gann's words, daring to voice the almost unsayable complexity. And then I read the social media comments. On a Facebook group, where the article was posted, I found glib hatred aimed at this loving mother, for her confession that she would have aborted if she had known.

A lot of people feel strongly about the abortion of 'abnormal' fetuses – either believing it's evil, or that taking away the right to abort is evil. The only thing I am sure of is my unwillingness to judge.

I support any woman's right to have screening and testing, to know as much as she would like, and to do with this information what she wants, whether it's just to prepare for a child with a disability, or not to continue with a pregnancy. And yet the evolving market for NIPT is increasingly commodified. Since 2017, private clinics have offered a simple maternal blood test to screen for a wildly disparate list of single-gene disorders, including Noonan's, achondroplasia (a common genetic cause of dwarfism), brittle bone disease and Rett syndrome.[38] A pregnant woman can book an NIPT test and scan 'for Down's syndrome and certain other genetic conditions' at her local branch of the maternity store Mothercare.[39] I find it disturbing that genetic screening can now be casually done, and I dislike the underlying assumption – that any genetic 'imperfection' is just a negative cross in a box. To give one example, prenatal DNA testing is now available for Klinefelter syndrome – a condition in which males have an extra X chromosome and have reduced testosterone and, often, infertility. It affects as many as one in 660 males and can be so mild many men don't even know they have it (according to the NHS website, 'most boys and men with Klinefelter syndrome will not be significantly affected and can live normal, healthy lives'[40]). But still, about half of women who get the diagnosis for their unborn child terminate the pregnancy.[41]

The sad fact is that families are attacked whatever their path. It's a cruel world online and there are no easy answers. Jane Fisher of ARC says that for women who speak up about terminating a Down's pregnancy, 'the vitriol and hate-mail are mind-boggling'. People with Down's have also long been targets. In the comments following one *Daily Mail* article about the modelling career of Natty, a beautiful girl with Down's syndrome, someone left a link to a site describing how to perform a 'post-birth abortion' and said this is what should have happened to Natty. You don't get hardened to such comments; Natty's mother, the disability rights campaigner Hayley Goleniowska told me, 'I have to go offline and cry.'

*

If someone with a new genetic diagnosis for their child asked me for advice, I'd say: the most important thing to understand is that it doesn't define them. Your child is still your child. You are still you. Life will feel normal again. No one person is likely to have everything on a list of symptoms. Physical difficulties are often treatable. And so are emotional and behavioural issues. Yes, a child with a genetic condition can, sometimes and sometimes not, have behavioural and social differences, a label that sounds very frightening out of context. But, again, she or he is your child, is wonderful, and you will love them and they will love you. Disruptive behaviour – if it happens, and even if it's worse than the difficult behaviour most children have in one way or another at some point – is just an island in the great world of that wonderfulness and love. Neurodiverse traits can be challenging, but they can also be strengths, even their own kind of genius. We don't yet have words to describe these different ways of seeing the world.

Like mine, Caroline White's initial shock turned to acceptance and happiness. When Caroline told me Seb's diagnosis story seven years after his birth, over cups of tea in her living room in the heart of the city of Bath, her three young children were playing on the floor. Dominic, then five, and two-year-old Polly didn't know there was anything different about their big brother (although Dominic had mentioned not long before that Seb 'speaks funny'). They were the picture of an ordinary, close, loving family. Seb and Polly were in cahoots about being naughty, while Dominic was quieter. Seb was a handsome, chuckly, witty, independent boy who had a habit of stealing strawberries from the fridge. He loved magic and sports and was quite the computer whizz. Within minutes of my arrival he had charmed his way into my mobile phone and as his mother and I talked, I caught glimpses of various apps and then my photo stream as he flicked through it with lightning speed (he was careful not to delete anything).

'When Seb was born, I assumed a lifetime of exclusion, feeling sad and second-rate – I dreaded the future,' Caroline told me. 'But after a while I realized he's not a list of characteristics in a textbook; he's my child. We lead a typical existence. Seb goes to school, plays football, goes to birthday parties. I'm excited to see where he goes with his life, what job he has, whether he has a relationship.'

Caroline had once assumed the sporty son she dreamed of had been taken away, but ended up realizing 'It was me taking it away – and in fact he is a sporty boy. And what matters is that he's happy and lives a full life.'

Today Caroline is chair of the Bath branch of learning disability charity Mencap and writes a popular blog on disability inclusion (forceofnature21.com). Caroline would give anything to have Seb's precious early weeks back to enjoy. She did enjoy him, of course, eventually. The turning point came one sunny day when the family were relaxing in the garden. Seb was four months old and, sitting in his colourful play-nest, he started to smile.

At that moment, Caroline saw him, truly saw him. Seb was so beautiful, he took her breath away. She took a photograph. She suddenly knew, then, that everything was going to be OK.

That was the first good day.

Hayley Goleniowska and her husband Bob had 'shrugged off' a one in 297 chance of their baby having Down's syndrome and the diagnosis was made shortly after the birth of their second daughter, Natty, with a distant formality: talk about leaflets, a poem that compared having a child with a disability to holidaying in Holland instead of Italy[†] and the comment

---

† This 1987 text, 'Welcome to Holland' by Emily Perl Kingsley, is one of the first things a parent of a child diagnosed with a disability is usually given. It explains that one has to adjust one's expectations of parenthood, from a glorious holiday in Italy to a drab one in Holland. Many like it, but I found it unhelpfully negative and still feel rebellious about it. If anything, I'd compare having a child with a disability to the wild adventure and thrills of being rerouted to the jungle.

that 'some of them even go to a mainstream school'. Hayley, a former teacher who had become a stay-at-home mother when her older daughter, Mia, was born, panicked, cried and 'wanted to scream'. A diagnosis of a rare genetic condition is isolating and uncertain. The diagnosis of a well-known and easily recognizable syndrome like Down's is hard because everyone has an idea of what it means already (albeit often an inaccurate one).

Today, Hayley, a glowing woman with a voice as soft as a flute, is one of Britain's most devoted campaigners for people with Down's syndrome and their families. Hayley's blog Downssideup.com, which gets 40,000 hits a month, has become a fulltime job. Blogs like Hayley's – and the proliferation of Facebook groups for families affected by syndromes – bring communities together, crowdsourcing grassroots knowledge on symptoms and traits which the medical profession still lacks.

In 2016, Hayley gave a speech to student nurses about Down's syndrome. Natty, then nine, with glossy brown hair and rosy cheeks, was in the audience. At the podium, Hayley choked back tears as she spoke about her fear at the time of diagnosis. 'Our youngest daughter Natalia was born on our bathroom floor. What followed is etched in my heart and frozen in time forever. The look of panic on the midwife's face. My brain dared not formulate a question because I was terrified of hearing what I thought was my worst nightmare. What I had been conditioned to fear. Our community midwife wept – and there was no need to be sorry . . . how I wish I could go back and relive that day knowing what I now know.'

Hayley turned to her daughter. 'Natty, I'm so sorry I got it wrong before I knew you,' she said, her voice breaking.

In tears, Hayley thanked the audience, and looked down – to find Natty had run from the audience to hug her on the stage. 'It's OK, Mum,' Natty said.

The nurses rose to their feet to applaud, tissues in every hand as they wiped tears from their eyes too.

With love, Natty forgave her mother. I hope Joel will forgive me, too.

7

'Mum'

'Nothing makes a woman out of a girl faster than coping
with a congenital defect in her child.'

EVERETT KOOP, ONE OF THE FIRST PAEDIATRIC SURGEONS[1]

Every day, we travelled to the hospital from East Finchley,
carrying bottles of my expressed milk, then left at night. As I
walked up the escalator at Warren Street station, then around
the corner towards UCH, I felt with every step a growing
magnetic pull towards my baby; then, when I entered his
ward, I was shut down by sadness at finding him in this lonely
place, being cared for by strangers, and having to leave him
there. At home, I set my alarm clock through the nights to
express milk for his tube feeds, while he lay in a plastic box,
having never tasted a drop.

The fact I couldn't just pick Joel up or lie next to him or
take him outside made him seem, sometimes, like a stranger.
The experiences Joel was undergoing, one after the other –
having a tube placed via his nose into his intestines; having a
drip inserted under his scalp because he had run out of other
veins; his heart failing – and then the diagnosis of a genetic
condition, and the prospect of major surgery – eventually
started to feel too much to take in.

In some of the worst moments, as I was holding Joel in the high dependency unit and crooning 'I Can Sing a Rainbow', my voice continued – outwardly performing the maternal role – while inside I didn't know what I was feeling. A tiny piece of me wasn't sure I wanted to be a mother any more and I felt this part of myself was unacceptable. I didn't realize that mothers could feel this way. I believed I was the only mother in the world who felt this, that I was the worst mother in the world. Grieving for my son, whom I was convinced I had failed and lost, I sat for hours as I held Joel in the neonatal unit's big reclining armchairs, wondering how I could magically rewind time and erase my fears; I even considered begging for a lobotomy. On the very worst morning, I dressed in silence in the dark; birds tweeting in the swelling light; the inevitability of another day. Every movement felt impossibly heavy. I looked out of the bedroom window and thought about whether I really could jump. Went into the bathroom, took a razor and ran it over my wrist, pressing lightly. I realized then how hard I would have to push to cut my wrist. I knew I could never actually do it. Teeth chattering, I walked downstairs, where Phil and my parents were waiting for me.

On the Tube into central London, every day for weeks, I thought of jumping under trains. I didn't want to be a bad mother. But I also didn't want to die. So I carried on, thinking weird morbid thoughts, like envying old people because they must have had happy lives not to have ended them.

Of course I sought help. The doctor who compared Joel's diagnosis with that of the child missing a finger wrote a letter summarizing everything I'd told her and sent it to the neonatal doctors. I only knew this because I found it in Joel's hospital notes, where it lay for all the nurses to read. I had assumed the doctor was a psychotherapist or counsellor who abided by rules of confidentiality, but when I complained, she explained (too late) she was a psychiatrist and always wrote detailed letters about her patients. I felt betrayed and ashamed. Now the neonatal staff would know I was a mother who couldn't cope.

I was referred to a psychologist on the NHS who was kind. Once a week we met at the top of a tall tower in Archway. My parents escorted me there, afraid to let me take the Tube alone. Every week the therapist asked me: 'How is Joel?' She explained that my anxiety and depression were a natural response to a traumatic experience.

Because I had lost all perspective, only after two months of this did I start to understand what she was saying, and something else also dawned on me. Loving mothers weren't perfect – it was normal to wish motherhood away at times.

I wasn't a bad mother, I was a good mother who in fact cared, if anything, so much I was making myself ill with guilt. And if adjustment to motherhood was difficult for all mothers, the pressures of the neonatal unit and a genetic diagnosis made it more intense. Gradually, over months and years, I forgave myself – completely.

If only I'd known from the start what I found out later: that almost everything I experienced emotionally in the neonatal unit is classic.

In the years after Joel came home, I made friends whose experiences, it turned out, mirrored my own. Women like Miranda, an academic at a top-tier university, who became alienated from those caring for her and her baby.

When Miranda found herself in a fetal medicine unit at the age of thirty-seven, she and her husband Stephen had already suffered a series of miscarriages and had conceived their baby with IVF treatment. A cervical suture was performed to strengthen the neck of Miranda's womb, to lessen the risk of miscarrying again. At the ultrasound scan to check the suture, the consultant fell quiet. Ushering Miranda and husband Stephen – also an academic – into another room, he said: 'There is a problem with this baby.'

Miranda and Stephen's baby had exomphalos major – a rare and serious condition in which organs develop outside the abdomen. In this case, the liver was ballooning outside the fetus, contained in a thin membrane, and would have to be sewn back into the body immediately after birth. What scared the couple more was that exomphalos can be associated with other conditions, including the serious chromosomal disorder Edwards' syndrome and major heart defects. Miranda and Stephen were told that because advances in fetal medicine that allow treatment for exomphalos are so recent, not that many children with exomphalos have survived. Many given the diagnosis in the past simply terminated their pregnancies. Now, an amniocentesis would tell Miranda and Stephen if the baby had a chromosomal condition like Edwards' syndrome, but the baby could only be assessed for the full range of genetic and heart conditions after birth.

As a researcher by nature and profession, it was the not knowing that upset Miranda most. Crying and in shock, she didn't want to sleep that night after the amniocentesis because she didn't want to endure that moment of waking up and forgetting about it, only to remember again. And her plans to buy baby clothes faded like a mirage.

A few days later, the consultant offered them a termination. 'We've never sewn in an abnormal baby before,' the consultant added. The casual harshness of the medical language shocked Miranda, as I was shocked to be told about my son being 'shunted' (the way the fetal medics described his shunt procedure) and, later, 'starved' (how surgical staff described nil by mouth before operations). Miranda's consultant meant that the cervical stitch would not have been done if the baby had a disability, presumably because its life would not be worth saving. 'How would you feel to have a severely handicapped child?' he asked Miranda. The medical student in the room started to cry. 'I don't know,' Miranda said.

They had tried so hard to have a baby and had thought if it had Down's syndrome they would keep it. But facing the reality of a child with disabilities, Miranda increasingly felt she wasn't strong enough to cope. 'I thought I'd crack up by the end of the pregnancy,' she told me, frankly, sitting on my sofa with a mug of tea one winter afternoon. Stephen was 'clear-headed' that there was no need to terminate, but Miranda wanted a termination. She was already feeling bereaved. Her mind was filled with thoughts of giving birth to a stillborn baby, or the baby dying a few days old. Like me, she also started researching adoption.

One possible outcome, Miranda was told, was that their baby – a boy, they now knew – might have giantism, which they were told can be associated with childhood cancers and 'retardation'. 'You'll still have a lovely baby; it's not the end of the world,' a midwife told Miranda. But for Miranda it was the end of her world. She felt deeply ashamed and guilty for thinking it, but it was 'petrifying' for two academics to adjust to the idea that their son might be 'retarded'. Or that he might dwarf them, as average-sized adults. 'It was hard to connect him with myself,' Miranda now reflects. 'But I felt I wasn't allowed to say that.'

Major heart defects were ruled out with further scans and Miranda committed to going through with the pregnancy. Induced at full term for the birth, Miranda walked, in early labour, through hospital corridors gazing at posters about different syndromes on the walls. She became convinced her son would have Kabuki syndrome, a rare, multi-system disorder.

But Saul – as they named him – didn't have Kabuki syndrome. Saul was delivered by a large team, and his liver was put back into his abdomen successfully. When Miranda met me, seven years after his birth, Saul was a little small for his age with slightly weak stomach muscles after his neonatal surgery, but otherwise a very well, happy boy living a totally normal life, with a healthy younger brother. None of the scary stuff had happened – nothing at all. But what still haunted Miranda was the way she felt in hospital, the way she – a high-risk 'case' – had lost all her power.

Having felt 'wrong-footed' by some doctors in the fetal medicine unit, Miranda had continued to feel this way in the neonatal unit, where Saul's hospital notes contained 'rude remarks' about her 'aggressive' way of speaking. She told me: 'They all loved Stephen, who joked with the nurses, while I was growling, feeling I was losing it completely.' It's important to note that Miranda is not by any stretch of the imagination unpleasant or belligerent. She is, in fact, an exceptionally polite character, and a deep-feeling one; at that time in hospital, she was anxious and depressed.

Some people cope in a hospital environment, becoming institutionalized; others never feel at ease. Stephen is especially sociable and easy-going, the type of person who can get along with absolutely anyone, while Miranda is warm and friendly but also sensitive, with what she describes as 'an obsessive personality'; she has suffered from depression in the past. Stephen, despite his field being the arts, instinctively grasped medical terminology and seemed to sail through hospital life, joking with the doctors and nurses. While he took the role of the 'front man', Miranda, numb with shock and unable to 'perform normality', felt cast as 'the emotional wreck' with a history of depression and obsessive compulsive disorder. One of the hospital staff wrote a letter to Miranda's GP saying he should 'watch her' because 'she seems very distressed and her mind keeps going around in loops'. The GP told her to pull herself together. Miranda was not in fact losing her mind, but an extremely bright, thoughtful woman having a natural and understandable response to being the mother of an ill baby. Yet she felt 'earmarked for complete breakdown' by medical staff. It was humiliating.

The relationship between mother and doctor in such extreme circumstances is one that can resonate long into the future. Years later, Miranda's second son started playing football. One of the neonatal consultants' husbands was the coach, and the interaction still felt awkward to Miranda. When, on the sidelines, the consultant said 'Hello, Miranda', Miranda imagined she could hear a patronizing note. Once, after such a conversation, Miranda asked her husband Stephen, 'Did I come across as normal?' He replied, 'What are you talking about? You just had a conversation as two mothers.' They were both mothers, and both professionals – they were technically equals. Rationally, Miranda realized the doctor's tone was in fact as friendly as ever, and that the doctor saw many former patients around the city, and that her own experience was probably just another case to the consultant. But somehow, even so long afterwards, Miranda worried she was, in some way, still being judged inferior for not having reacted in the happiest, calmest possible way to her child's hospital nightmare.

I asked Rebecca Chilvers, the lead neonatal unit psychologist at Guy's and St Thomas's Hospital, about the typical issues neonatal mothers go through. Her response was essentially a tick list of the experiences of mothers like Miranda and me. (I've focused on mothers, but of course there is also a classic experience for fathers which is difficult in a different way. As Rebecca Chilvers reminded me, fathers are the ones who witness delivery and 'they sometimes find it hard to ask for help, and often feel like they're carrying a sense of responsibility for everything, looking after their partners, keeping the family home running, looking after the other children . . . they have to be strong.')

First, the unnatural separation of a mother and her baby affects everyone. My strong and capable psychotherapist friend Eve was discharged from hospital the day after giving birth to her twins. Amber had died at birth, and Noah was in intensive care. For Eve, the separation she endured was 'barbaric'.

One of the memories which has stuck in Eve's mind is how hard it was to leave Noah in the care of a nurse she didn't feel comfortable with. At eight o'clock one evening, while Eve was holding Noah, a nurse muttered aloud: 'It's too quiet tonight. I know something awful's going to happen.' The nurse started to put Noah back in his cot and Eve thought she pulled his arm in an uncomfortable way. Eve couldn't leave Noah alone with this nurse, she thought – so she spent the whole night sitting in a chair next to him.

As long ago as the 1890s, doctors knew that dividing mothers and sick babies was a bad idea. In *fin de siècle* France when the first incubators came into use, the visionary early neonatologist Pierre Budin observed, 'mothers, separated from their infants, soon lost all interest in those whom they were unable to nurse or cherish. It is better by far to put the little one in an incubator by its mother's bedside. The supervision which she exercises is not to be lightly estimated . . . if the nurse be negligent, the mother does not fail to remark that the incubator is being allowed to grow cold.' He added that among mothers who were unable to feed their babies themselves: 'I have been grieved to see a certain number of women come more and more rarely to visit their child, and gradually lose all interest in it.'[2] When these mothers were notified that their babies were well and about to be discharged, they made no response, and Budin was forced to hand over the infants to a home for abandoned children. (Later, in the mid-twentieth century at CHOP's pioneering NICU, nurses would sometimes offer to adopt abandoned babies.[3]) Budin calculated the percentage of mothers who abandoned their babies in hospital was as high as 28 per cent, a figure he considered 'sad in the extreme'. For this reason, he insisted that neonatal care must be not only about saving the baby's life but also establishing breastfeeding.[4]

Today, any decent neonatologist would agree that the mother should be allowed to sleep next to her baby (if she wants to) – comfortably, not dozing in an upright chair – as much as possible, even when the baby is critically ill. The fact almost none have this privilege in the modern high-tech neonatal ward isn't a failure of doctors and nurses – it comes down, at least in the NHS, to lack of money to build a modern unit where a large number of mothers could 'room in'.

The second experience many mothers share – and closely linked to mothers' separation from their babies – is the difficulty of expressing milk. In the first neonatal hospitals, wet nurses were employed to live in dormitories on the wards. In late nineteenth-century France, wrote Pierre Budin, the wet nurses 'should be allowed to keep their own infants, for if they suckled only puny little beings, who are sometimes scarcely able even to swallow, their milk would diminish and even disappear'.⁵ The wet nurses had their work cut out: in October 1895, Budin noted, his *maternité* hospital had fourteen wet nurses for fifty 'weaklings'. Including feeding their own babies, then, each wet nurse had to keep as many as five babies nourished – giving as many as forty feeds every day.⁶

By the 1920s, wet nurses were still used, but the Chicago neonatologist Julius Hess was recommending mothers of premature babies should express their milk, either by hand or using vacuum breast pumps. The inventive physician devised hand-operated pumps which allowed a mother to express milk directly into a flask with a stopper to keep the milk free from contamination.⁷ Electric breast pumps followed soon after. Breast milk banks quickly came into use, too, so mothers who had extra milk could donate it for babies in hospital. In 1940s Birmingham, milk donors were paid two pence per ounce.⁸ Today, donor breast milk is still vital for the most fragile babies whose own mothers can't produce enough of their own milk – and expressing is a way of life for NICU mothers. But it's not simple.

Having become a mother at twenty-three weeks, it was hard for the ever-capable Eve to get any milk, and she felt she was 'failing dismally . . . everyone would be sitting there with bottles and I'd be sitting there with a syringe, and I would get, if I was lucky, on a good day, 2 millilitres.' Even if you don't have physical trouble lactating, the round-the-clock regime is not easy when you are separated from your baby. It's one thing with a healthy baby to be woken in the night, but when your baby is a little body you've hardly ever touched, in a little box miles away, it feels unnatural to set the alarm for 2 a.m.

When Joel was a couple of days old, the nurse looking after him took me to the little expressing room and showed me how to squeeze out impossibly scarce amounts of colostrum.

Quickly the amounts requested of me grew and the hospital loaned me an industrial-strength expressing machine to use at home. I followed the advice to the letter. But there was a problem. I didn't have enough milk. The nurses tell you to look at a photo of the baby while you express, but that just made me sad – it reminded me I could only 'feed' Joel by touching a photo.

The pressure to breastfeed or express as part of being a 'good mother' is something many women feel and which causes a great deal of sleep deprivation and stress, but when your baby is sick, all this is multiplied. It requires superhuman stamina to pump the recommended six to eight number of times a day while also looking after your baby in a neonatal unit for months. My expressing sessions lasted for as long as an hour at a time, sometimes more, because it took that long to get 30 or 40 millilitres. I set my alarm clock for a few hours after I'd gone to sleep and pumped for an hour in the middle of the night while watching TV, then washed and sterilized the equipment. In the hospital, I spent hour after hour in the expressing room where the unit mothers expressed, talked and cried. And still I felt a failure.

My feelings weren't always virtuous. Once in the expressing room I met a mother I'd never seen before. She was visiting the hospital for a check-up and had nipped into the room to breastfeed *a real baby*, not express. How bizarre. Here we all were expressing, and yet until this moment there had never been a baby in sight. I wanted to like the mother but jealousy got in the way. In her pity for me I felt a wall between us; I couldn't help imagining this woman's life, how she was free to take her baby to the park that sunny afternoon.

When it became clear I was not producing enough milk, I started expressing even more often. I began a new expressing session every two and a half hours in the day and every three to four hours overnight. Given that I was expressing for at least forty-five minutes at each session, I was now spending a large proportion of my life pumping. There was hardly time to eat or sleep. This sleep-deprivation meant I didn't even realize how tired I was, and I felt more separated from my baby than ever. I tried wheeling the pump into the ward so I could express next to Joel's incubator, but even with a screen around me, it felt too public, and this lack of privacy affected my milk even more. So the milk didn't flow, and with an alternative remedy, flax seeds, not helping either, I was prescribed the maximum dose of a drug called Domperidone. This is a medicine which speeds up the gut, but mothers of babies in neonatal care have sometimes been given it off-licence, solely for the side effect of increasing lactation.† It had little effect, but I took it for months. Meanwhile what I had for Joel was supplemented with donated milk from other mothers. (The most vulnerable babies in the NICU are usually fed with breast milk, not formula.) I was grateful but also envied their endless effortless bottlefuls.

Gradually I gave up on the punishing expressing routine. I started to express only two or three times a day and let myself sleep through the night. As we prepared for Joel to come home in his fifth month, I made the decision to stop expressing altogether. The less I expressed, the happier and stronger I became. It was only later that I found out others had chosen

---

† A practice no longer recommended; Domperidone has since been banned in the USA and concerns have been raised about its side effects, from serious cardiac risks to the baby to a small number of reports of psychological problems for the mother, despite the fact that Domperidone is not thought to cross the blood–brain barrier. I had started taking a high dose of Domperidone two or three days before my own anxiety and depression started, which has made me wonder.

not to express at all while their baby was in neonatal care, and that the doctors and nurses had accepted it. I could have done the same, but it had never occurred to me.

The third thing mothers go through in the neonatal unit is the public scrutiny. One mother told me of the feeling she had, looking at her baby in the incubator: 'It's almost like it's not your baby.' It's weird for any woman being suddenly referred to by hospital midwives solely as 'mum' – there's a loss of the identity you had before – but when you're in the neonatal unit reading about yourself as 'mum' in your baby's notes, with comments on how 'mum' is managing and recording that you held 'baby' for forty-five minutes or how many bottles of milk you expressed, the guilt and pressure any new mother feels is – again – magnified. Nurses, midwives and doctors, of course, might well argue that they cannot be expected to remember everyone's names. But calling a mother by her name, affirming her individuality and identity in such a small and subtle way, could help avoid antenatal and postnatal depression, which is especially likely to affect the mother of a baby who is sick.

Mothers of healthy babies can work out their own way of mothering in the privacy of their own home. In the neonatal unit, you're learning, and making mistakes, in public. I couldn't help comparing myself with the others, like another mother in the high dependency unit who was only in her early twenties and looked after her baby Jonny beautifully. If someone else stayed later at night than me or was already there in the morning when I came in, I felt pangs of shame. When researching for this book, years after Joel came out of hospital, I returned to look up his old medical notes. All that time later I still couldn't bring myself to read the medical staff's observations about me in the file. Here I was now, a writer, also working as an editor for the government's website in West-minster part-time, a fully functioning member of society. But on some level, I still could taste – and fear – the powerlessness I once had as a 'new mum' who couldn't cope.

Every morning when I saw Joel, the first thing I'd do after gazing at him and holding his fingers through the incubator porthole would be to read through his ever-growing notes and then tidy up his corner. I was quite rigid when it came to how I wanted Joel's nursing station and cupboard to be arranged. If any nurse tried to reorganize by, say, putting his nappies in his sleepsuit drawer, God help them. But the matron under-stood that this was the only control I had, the only bit of mothering I could do. She told a nurse who'd tried to repos-ition his belongings: 'She's the mum and she decides where things go. We're just babysitting for her.' At home, a new mother gets to play with a whole nursery and move her baby wherever she wants to take it. In hospital, for a nurse to try to fold my baby's clothes more neatly seemed a criticism; it infringed in some way on my motherhood. And there was so little I could do to assert my motherhood in the unit.

Once, a lovely, kind neonatal consultant remarked to me that she had observed how when a sick baby is born, it's difficult for parents to see it as their baby. She had always remembered one mother who, on seeing her baby for the first time in the neonatal unit, said to him: 'You are the most beau-tiful thing I've ever seen.' That's rare, the consultant told me. I saw it all differently. I told her that the other parents who were silent were probably also thinking their child was the most beautiful thing they had ever seen, but felt too self-conscious to say words like those out loud in public, overheard by a nurse and a doctor. A mother who takes her baby home can talk to her without being observed and overheard. The neonatal unit mother has no such privacy. She can feel inhibited and unable to express herself. To me it felt like constant stage fright – being in the spotlight.

My friend, the intelligent and sensitive Allie, whose twins were born at twenty-five weeks, sees herself as a 'self-contained' person. That time in the neonatal units where she ended up spending the first ten months after birth felt, to her, 'like going through the wardrobe door' and disappearing from the world. Like me, she didn't reach out to other people, either in the unit or among her friends: she had no energy left for anyone else. Allie once gave me one of the best descriptions of motherhood in the neonatal unit I have ever heard. 'I was focused on trying to be what was expected of me,' she said. She was 'trying to be a good mum in extremely odd circumstances, and being a good mum in those circumstances is sitting next to an incubator for hours.' But the reality? 'I was not bonding with my children at all. I didn't know they were going to make it, so how can you bond?'

In this weird, highly controlled space where you have to get permission to go anywhere and do anything, Allie felt 'very limited'. The publicness of the space affected her strongly. 'Beth was four months old when I first held her with no one else in the room – you are always under the eye of nurses or doctors, and you're trying to be with your child when you don't know how to be with your child. You're being watched all the time. So bonding with your child is almost impossible.'

She felt she was being judged, she told me. We talked in the pub one night about how this guilty feeling is really self-judgement because the doctors and nurses are too busy to judge. Yet, like me, Allie compared herself constantly to other unit parents. She would leave in the evening to eat, and some parents would still be in the unit after twelve hours – 'and I'd be like, oh my God, I'm so bad'. One can keep up a regime of sitting around the clock by the incubator for weeks, but when your child is in hospital for months not weeks, it's hard to sustain. Allie tried to be there as much as she could, but still felt she had failed, 'because there were always mums who'd been there more than me, who slept there and never left'.

I have always remembered the constantly high, happy mother whose relatively well baby spent just a few days in the high dependency unit and who, before bouncing home, told the long-stay parents she had never been parted from any of her children for even five minutes. Only in the unit a short time, either she or her husband was with her baby 24/7. That mother broke my heart one day as we were eating a swift lunch in the unit together, perched on chairs in the waiting room. 'Aw, poor Joel,' she said. 'Did you know Joel cries sometimes late at night? And you know, sometimes the nurses don't go to him right away. I feel *so* sorry for him.'

Even the global organization promoting 'family integrated care' – a positive protocol aimed at making NICU parents feel part of their baby's care and reducing stress all round – perhaps fails to understand fully what it's like to be a NICU parent. I was stunned to see that one of its posters put up in neonatal units goes so far as to suggest a timetable of a typical day for a parent, specifying what they could – which a vulnerable mother may read as *should* – be doing during every part of the day and night. The timetable included pumping breast milk and doing feeds around the clock, a bizarre mention of exercise time when not at the hospital (because of course NICU mothers have the spare time and energy to work out!), what time they should arrive at the unit in the morning (8–10 a.m.) and a list of tasks to achieve during the morning and afternoon. Of course the timetable is not meant to be prescriptive and bossy, but it read to me like another set of expectations pushed on already over-burdened mothers.

The feeling that there is a parent who is doing more than you is an illusion of maternal guilt often experienced, ironically, by the most dutiful. When I returned to the neonatal unit six years later to observe, I was struck by how, in fact, few parents visited their children. Across three full days I spent in neonatal intensive care, I saw only two or three babies out of twelve have their parents or grandparents visit. In high dependency, parents were typically coming in sometime during the day, perhaps after lunch to be with their baby for a few hours. A parent's time is pulled in different directions by the need to express, by older children at home, by the need to eat and rest. Mothers are usually on maternity leave but fathers typically need to continue working. It sounds easy to sit by an incubator for hours, but anyone who has done it will tell you that it's not. Other than holding your baby (when you're finally able to – and even then there is a limit to how many hours one can sit in a chair holding a baby – you can't even walk around the room with them), there is very little you can actually do. As Allie put it to me, 'You're just bearing witness to a medical situation. You're watching something unfold and you have very little role to play.'

Hospital life can be oddly boring. As weeks turned into months, I got into the habit of regularly wiping down the outside of Joel's incubator and its drawers, the wheeled nursing station which held his bulging notes, and his cubicle where we stored his clothes. It sounds silly – these things were regularly cleaned by hospital staff and already shiny – but I picked up this activity from the other mothers. Many of us did it. It was something we could do to fill those long hours sitting next to our sleeping babies.

Perhaps it also had something to do with a fourth common experience: anxiety around hygiene. Like me, Eve became, as she puts it, a 'hand-washing militant'. The daunting responsibility of becoming a mother for the first time is tough for almost everyone, but when your baby is very ill, you are not just responsible for an ordinarily vulnerable baby, but for a baby who might die. The overwhelming fears any new mother experiences about something bad happening to her baby are not paranoia in the neonatal unit. When Joel was born, it was flu season, babies had died, and visitors were now limited. My sister flew in to meet her nephew but she wasn't allowed to see him. There were signs warning any visitors to stay away if they had been ill, which I took literally. I became paranoid about going near Joel that winter, when I'd just stepped off a Tube filled with sneezing, coughing people. Suddenly I was facing dilemmas – was my nose sniffly enough to be a cold? Should I go into the unit with my possible germs at all?

The institutionalized obsessive compulsive disorder over hygiene played a major role in the constant guilt I felt. Just how rigorous do I need to be to keep Joel safe, I used to wonder? What was enough? I followed the rules about cleaning my breast pump to the letter, washing the flanges and tubes in hot soapy water. Following the instruction literally that the water should be 'as hot as you can bear', I scalded myself repeatedly as I sought to find the limit of what I could endure. I ran tubing through the sterilizer at 2, 3 and 4 a.m.; laid things out to dry on spotless virgin kitchen towel. If I brushed part of the tubing with unsterilized hands, I washed and sterilized it again. I didn't allow myself to express in bed in the middle of the night; I had to go downstairs so I could go through the careful sterilizing procedure fully alert. Should I be wiping Joel's incubator down with antiseptic wipes, and if so, should it be daily? Should I wipe down the exterior as well as interior of the pink cooler bag in which I brought my expressed milk to hospital? I once spent fifteen minutes in the unit toilet scrubbing the cooler bag after someone on the Tube coughed over it. Sometimes I would also babywipe my closed bottles of expressed milk, or even throw the contents away if I had sneezed while screwing on the lid or touched my breast with an unwashed hand while expressing. Later I learned psychologists call this hyper-vigilance and it's increasingly recognized as a common reaction to the constant panic of having a NICU baby.

It was only when I found myself wondering about how I could sterilize the sterilizer *itself* one day that I realized all this had to stop. I was much reassured by Giles Kendall explaining to me that in fact sterilizing was not necessary if you washed feeding things in hot water – and it didn't even have to be scalding, just as hot as felt *comfortable*. The top rack of the dishwasher would be fine, he told me. This was some of the happiest, most life-changing advice I had. From that sane day on, the sterilizer was unused and became positively dusty.

Seven years later, when I interviewed Eve, she talked about 'that smell' of the hospital handwash and hand sanitizer, which for NICU mothers conjures such strong feelings every time we enter a hospital and catch the scent again. 'It just takes me right back – it's almost like a flashback,' she told me.

Eve has also experienced a more traumatic kind of flashback. It started a year after Noah came home and lasted for three more years. She would be sitting anywhere – on a bus or in a queue – and she would suddenly hear the beeping of hospital monitors. The sound was so clear that she would turn around, startled, to look for the source. 'It would shake me out of my reality,' she said.

It took Eve some time to realize what was happening. She, like many others who have had similar experiences of parenting ill children in hospital, was suffering from post-traumatic stress disorder (PTSD).

I think Allie may have PTSD too. The neonatal experience left her with 'a real feeling of inadequacy'. She described her thoughts to me: 'I couldn't get pregnant; when we did, it didn't work; I didn't ever feel that I was pregnant. My children are born of science. I felt like I wasn't doing anything when they were born; I wasn't able to be a mum to them.'

It was only well after the girls had come home that Allie began to feel like a mother. Even when I met her – and the twins were six – she still confessed to me that privately she felt 'that my whole experience of having children is a failure. We still find it hard to call each other Mum and Dad. We do now, but it's taken us a long time, because we felt superfluous to our own experience.' You'd never guess these hidden thoughts, if you met Allie. She's a bright, kind, energetic (and as you can tell, highly articulate) woman with a high-flying career; a devoted mother to her twins. She's the kind of woman I'd have looked at in the neonatal unit, compared myself to, and found myself wanting.

There are common thoughts a NICU mother finds it shameful to say out loud, Rebecca Chilvers told me. Seeing her, parents finally get 'permission to say the unspeakable'. She sees parents 'agonizing over decisions that are hard to talk to friends and family about – whether they ought to have had a termination; wishing for a baby's suffering to end and for them to die and be at peace. Asking whether what they are doing in consenting to aggressive intensive care is the right thing, whether keeping a baby alive who will have life-long disabilities is the right thing.' She also sees 'resentment and jealousy towards parents of healthy babies – which is also very difficult to talk about with others for fear of judgement'. Chilvers added: 'It's important to help parents understand that they aren't "going crazy" or "losing their mind" but that their reactions are understandable in the context of such challenging circumstances.'

Antenatal and postnatal depression, OCD, anxiety, panic disorder, PTSD . . . Fetal medicine centres and neonatal units are barely starting to wake up to the need for specialist support for the parents whose babies' lives are in their hands.

*

Seven years after Joel's birth, I flew to Stockholm, Sweden, to see a very different NICU experience. It was spring in England, but the snow was still thick on the ground at the Karolinska Hospital at Solna, where many of the most premature and sick babies in Sweden are treated. In this progressive country, groundbreaking hospital architecture powerfully changes the course of health and mental health.

The shiny new neonatal unit at the *sjukhuis* (sickhouse, or hospital), and its linked units around the city at Huddinge and Danderyd, were designed to eliminate the unnatural separation between mothers and babies which occurs in the vast majority of neonatal units around the developed world.

To people here, it is all so obvious. Parent and newborn should be together, and so it happens, even in intensive care, with twenty-two-week-old babies on ventilators. Each incubator is in what they call a 'pod' – a room with a bed for a parent. There are four pods in each large-windowed ward – one in each corner – and the space in the middle is the nursing station. The walls of each pod are formed of sliding doors, which are opened and closed, balancing the needs for family privacy and medical monitoring. Each pod can be almost completely closed off apart from a doorway-sized entrance for a nurse or doctor, and even this can be covered with a screen, so the family have their own space. The mother comes here immediately after delivering her baby and her postnatal care is done in the pod – in tandem with her baby's treatment. Yes, this really is intensive care.

As if this wasn't enough, each baby's parents are also given a completely private double bedroom (with wooden beds, flat-screen TV and an ensuite) on the ward, just steps away from the pod, so they can get more rest, since the intensive care environment is inevitably quite disturbed. With these two places to sleep, there is no need to go home at all, unless you want to, or have other children, in which case mothers and fathers and grandparents typically take turns to stay at the hospital. Once the baby is off CPAP, it is moved into the bedroom. These private rooms have monitors for the baby's vital signs, which the medical staff can see on screens outside the room; there are also beepers which alert nurses if the baby's heart rate gets too high.

For staff and parents alike here, the way other countries do neonatal care is bemusing. When I explained to them that (with one exception, the night before his first operation at Great Ormond Street Hospital), I didn't get to spend all night in a bed next to Joel for almost five months, until I 'roomed in' for the last few nights of his special care before he came home, everyone looked shocked. Even when Joel went to Great Ormond Street, after his operation there was just a reclining chair in the ward for me to sit in, and I felt very lucky to be given a basic bedroom shared with another mother a five-minute walk away in the nurses' accommodation. Just these nights of slight proximity – and the few nights I was allowed before Joel's discharge from UCH in a room a floor above his ward – were healing for me; I got to know Joel by hearing his little breaths late at night; I felt safer and less weirdly disconnected knowing he was near. How transformed would the whole experience have been for me if I could have slept comfortably beside Joel throughout?

I asked the premature baby charity Bliss if there were any neonatal units in Britain where parents could sleep next to their baby, but they were only aware of one (in north London). Even there, the parent can only stay with their child in special care. There are very few equivalents to the Swedish intensive care and high dependency model in the world outside Scandinavia, but more and more hospitals are consulting the Karolinska on how to replicate what they do. This is definitely the future. In the NHS, the problem is not that neonatologists don't agree with the Karolinska approach – they revere it. The problem is that hospitals have to be redesigned with rooms for parents in the neonatal wards, which is of course expensive, and the need for more space for parents would limit the numbers of inpatients.

For nurse Siri Lilliesköld, who has worked at the Karolinska since 2003 and helped launch this style of neonatal care in Sweden, there is a bizarre distinction in typical hospitals between the treatment of neonates and slightly older children. 'If you came to hospital with a one-, two-, three-year-old, you wouldn't leave them and go home,' she stressed to me over Swedish meatballs in the hospital canteen. But it's 'really odd', she said, that most parents of babies in neonatal units have to sleep outside the hospital. 'The infant needs its parents, we have to be honest.' The youthful and intelligent Siri, herself a mother who gave birth at Danderyd, was drawn to neonatal nursing for its 'existential' quality, she confided seriously as we walked down the hospital corridors. She started her nursing work with hospice patients, and then moved to neonatology, this field of birth and death. 'The questions one deals with at the beginning and the end of life . . . I just like to be there,' she said. She sees herself as a 'humanist', she explained, interested in 'the merging of the big questions we all carry – the meaning of life and death; the most important questions in our life – with very individualized care. We have to meet the essence of that person.'

The Karolinska's approach is an advanced interpretation of two person-centred philosophies which are increasingly popular in neonatal units around the world: NIDCAP (which stands for Newborn Individualized Developmental Care and Assessment Program) and Family Integrated Care. Both models are about bringing back the human touch to the neonatal unit. They aim to take care of the whole family, emotionally as well as physically, a practice which helps the child recover faster and better, and is also better for the parents.

For instance, if a parent feels their baby is behaving unusually, or wants to wait until the baby is calmer before starting a procedure, a nurse will take their input seriously. Procedures are often done with a parent holding and comforting the baby – premature babies are especially sensitive to pain, but being held skin-to-skin has a pain-relieving effect. Parents are encouraged to have as much 'kangaroo care' time (cuddling their baby skin-to-skin) as possible and to be with their baby as much as they can. At the Karolinska, a baby is often stabilized in the delivery room and the mother can also hold it immediately after birth. If the baby needs CPAP, instead of putting it in an incubator, the father may 'wear' the baby in a stretchy tube top – the CPAP machine is put on wheels beside him. The baby's breathing is much better as a result, Siri told me.

The parents – as opposed to a doctor or nurse – are seen as the baby's 'primary caregivers', even in intensive care, at the Karolinska. Of course medical staff still need to do their job – they monitor the babies and perform procedures like putting in cannulas and giving medication – but the parent is expected to do all the baby's 'cares', which in other countries remain typically the responsibility of nurses, albeit helped by parents. So the parents are the ones taking temperatures, weighing, giving tube feeds, checking the feeding tube is in the right place, filling in a nursing chart. 'Of course the medical responsibility is still on us,' Siri told me, 'but [nurses] go from task-oriented care to relationship-based care . . . they become less the doer and more good at coaching and empowering the parents.'

It took a while for modern sophisticated neonatal units with their high-tech equipment and procedures to learn that, ironically, a holistic, humane approach that costs nothing and uses no technology is just as crucial.

Take another simple but revolutionary idea that developed in parallel with NIDCAP. In Colombia, in 1978, the paediatrician Edgar Rey was facing a crisis: 30,000 babies a year were delivered at the Instituto Materno Infantil, the children of the poorest citizens of Bogotá, who lived in mountain shacks. The unit was so crowded that three babies shared each incubator, often infecting one another. More and more babies were dying. Desperate for some solution, Rey chanced across a paper about kangaroos, which mentioned how newborn joeys are tiny and immature, like a premature human. In the mother's pouch, a joey's body temperature is regulated by skin-to-skin contact and, breastfed, it grows until it's strong enough to hop out.

Such a simple idea; such a natural one. Rey told the mothers of premature babies at the institute to cuddle them skin-to-skin, twenty-four hours a day, frequently breastfeeding, just like kangaroos do. And it worked. Death and infection rates dropped.[9] Kangaroo mother care, as it became called, was picked up by hospitals in low-income countries: Venezuela, Brazil, Ethiopia, Madagascar, India, Cameroon. These days it's become a mainstay of every neonatal unit, strongly associated with better outcomes for babies (and mothers' mental health too).[10] And along with NIDCAP, Family Integrated Care, the practice in which parents stay with their babies and do most of their cares, is slowly spreading around the developed world.[11]

The neonatal unit has moved full circle and today the trend is to remember the most obvious, basic thing which, in the early days of paediatrics, was sometimes sidelined: the power of a mother's connection with her baby.

The atmosphere at the Karolinska hospitals seemed extraordinarily good. I spent most of my time at the Danderyd branch – Stockholm's major maternity hospital, which offers high dependency and special care – and I could not get over how unstressed the doctors and nurses appeared. There was none of the 'edge' I had experienced in other hospitals. When I saw the neonatal staffroom at this public hospital, I understood a little. It was straight out of an IKEA catalogue and unlike anything I have ever seen in the NHS or America. A long blond-wood table surrounded by cushioned chairs stood in the spotless room; large windows framed a fairy tale of falling snow. There was a large Samsung TV, a fancy coffee machine with stacks of pastel coffee cups neatly arranged on wooden shelving. Nurses, many wearing pretty clogs, sat on a modernist lime-green corner sofa and easy chairs, a beautiful ceramic dish filled with apples on a flowered doily resting on the coffee table in front of them. The walls were covered in a tasteful mural, and nurses could keep an eye on the vital signs of babies on several screens.

The parents seemed as happy and relaxed as the staff. In one private room, I watched as a young couple, Anna and John, cared for their daughter Matilda, their first child, born at thirty-two weeks. Matilda was well enough to stay with her parents in this room, in a cot next to their double bed. Here, Anna could use her breast pump in peace and privacy, and try to breastfeed Matilda very comfortably on the bed. Anna seemed shocked to hear my own story of separation from Joel. She and John were doing all Matilda's caring. They needed no permission to pick her up for a cuddle or a nuzzle; when they needed help, a nurse could come and give it. Anna worked in human resources; John in the army. They didn't have to worry about taking time off – their time at the hospital was covered by special pay for having a sick child, and then after Matilda came home, between them they were entitled to well over a year of paid leave on 90 per cent of their salaries.

*

I would have liked, in this book, to write more about the 'mothers' of fetal or neonatal medicine, but there seem only to be 'fathers'. For branches of medicine which treat the most intimate zones of the female body, fetal medicine, obstetrics and gynaecology have an oddly male, paternalistic history; the vast majority of acknowledged leaders of the field – for example, all the superstar names in fetal medicine at the time of writing – have been men. In science and medicine, as in other intensely time-demanding professions in which one sacrifices any personal life, it's harder for women to rise to the top, partly because many are not only doctors and scientists but mothers. We will see in the next chapter how one rare female surgeon had to dash to a park near the hospital where she worked to hand over her expressed breast milk to her husband and baby. And history too often fails to give pioneering women's achievements due notice – Google the trailblazing neonatologist Victoria Mary Crosse or the paediatrician Victoria Smallpeice, who ended the practice of starving premature babies, and you'll find the mentions of their names disappear by the second or third page of search results. Even those who are celebrated a little more, like Alice Stewart, the scientist who exposed the dangers of X-ray, or Mary Ellen Avery, who discovered surfactant, the substance babies need to breathe at birth, are not household names.

Medical history books and manuals of medicine also too often leave out the other female experience: that of the patients, the mothers. The usual focus is almost exclusively on the work of the (usually male) medics who have created these new forms of medicine – there is scant published information on what it's like for the women whose bodies have taught the doctors everything. As the historian Ann Dally wrote in her history of female surgery, *Women under the Knife*, 'much of the written history of gynaecology has been produced by gynaecologists, with themselves as heroes'.[12] The practice of midwifery has a strong female tradition, but in the 1700s, as obstetrics became increasingly technologized with the invention and manufacture of forceps and speculums, according to the feminist critic Karen Newman, 'obstetrics became professionalised and, ultimately, the province of men, especially among urban elites'.[13] She writes of 'the frequently horrific damage' instruments like forceps, speculums and obstetrical hooks could inflict on fetus and mother alike and their phallic shapes 'produced by a male-dominated technology linked to the growing status of obstetrics'.[14]

Even today, some fetal and obstetric doctors have a reputation among patients as somewhat 'macho'. One mother who underwent fetal procedures told me her male doctors didn't discuss her medical situation with her; only talking with her husband – which she felt was patriarchal, but she had to accept. The fetal doctors' tone felt, to this mother, 'business-oriented, matter-of-fact'. She cried in front of them but didn't feel she could share her feelings with them.

A strange gap seems to persist – a gap between the doctors and the mothers. As soon as Sophie, the doctor who endured so many procedures for her son Michael's congenital diaphragmatic hernia, gave birth, the family's contact with the fetal medics ended abruptly. This seems a common experience, and one which strikes families as odd. In the years since her time at the fetal medicine unit ended, Sophie has wanted to return to the hospital to see the consultant who did the operations. 'There's a bit of closure that hasn't happened,' she feels. 'Just to express gratitude, and to let them know what we've come through.' For the doctors to meet Michael, she says, 'would certainly mean something to me; I don't know how they would feel about it. They are good-hearted people, but so busy. It's such a collision of worlds: the worst thing that's ever happened in my life colliding with the doctors' day-to-day work, dealing with numerous heartbreaking situations. I have it too, in my own field, when I have to break the news of diagnoses. If I couldn't see the collision as a doctor myself, I'd think the fetal doctors could appear cold. But they've got to be businesslike to get through the work and help their patients.'

Did the fetal doctors respect you as a fellow doctor? I asked Sophie.

'I don't think they were fazed by the fact that I was a doctor, because I wasn't in doctor mode,' she said. 'From my doctor-y side, I was a little embarrassed at the time that I was handling it all so badly. But we're all levelled in this kind of situation – I became just a terrified, shaking, blubbering mother, which they're very used to dealing with.'

The doctors have mothers' and babies' best interests firmly in mind, yet the experience of the mother and baby somehow eludes them, is not recorded in the scientific papers. One could argue, why should it be? Her emotions are not considered part of the medical facts, any more than the feelings of an animal experimented on in the name of science are recorded.

When they were expecting their twins, my therapist friend Eve and her husband David sought a second opinion at another fetal medicine centre, where after hours of waiting, the 'icy, matter-of-fact' consultant had, Eve recalled to me, 'the most unpleasant, brusque bedside manner'. The doctor starkly explained that they faced the decision of whether to 'reduce' the pregnancy by terminating the ill twin. Such an invasive procedure would risk losing both babies, but it could also give the healthy fetus a better chance because the ill baby's condition could lead to polyhydramnios – the same excess of amniotic fluid I had, which can precipitate premature birth. Keeping going with the twin pregnancy would also mean Eve would have to carry to term, and finally give birth to, a baby who would die within hours. In a throwaway comment, made without eye contact, the doctor said: 'If you've got a problem with that, discuss it with a psychologist, not me.'

Eve, aged forty-one at the time of her pregnancy, is seen by her friends as a 'mother hen' who knows how to deal with everything. She is, by her own description, 'not backward in coming forward' – but in that moment in the clinic she felt extremely vulnerable and couldn't say a word in response. 'You've been poked and prodded in internal and external exams – I felt like a battery-farmed pregnant cow,' she told me.

In many cases (including my own), although a fetus is critically ill, the mother herself has no physical illness. But psychologically, she does need to be looked after; she herself is a high-risk case too.

Did fetal medicine reduce the status of mothers to that of a 'fetal incubator'? The health and rights of the unborn baby, made hyper-real through scanning, are taken seriously, but the mother's feelings are, sometimes, not considered. Doctors like Sophie's and Eve's almost certainly do not feel casual about their work, but can appear almost dismissive in the way they see cases.

The fetus is an individual with human rights – and yet many other mothers have, at times, felt oddly 'missing' – insignificant – in relation to their sick babies, both before and after their birth. The mother is reduced to the vessel holding the all-important baby, no longer a person with feelings and thoughts that matter or might be different to the norm – just like all the other 'mums' on the conveyor belt.

8

Operation

'Doctors do have favourite patients . . . I don't care too much for pretty hearts – give me someone who has been through some shit.'

KATE BULL, PAEDIATRIC HEART SURGEON[1]

For Joel, surgery started with that nursery-age idea, the 'tummy'. It's one of the first parts of the body a toddler becomes aware of, and chuckles about – a big, soft, cuddly, rather silly and ticklish place, normally warmed and comforted with milk. One of the first things that happened in Joel's life was that this innocent part of his body was to be cut into and rearranged.

A lot of babies have reflux – they vomit up milk and the acid indigestion makes them uncomfortable. Joel's reflux was on an extreme scale. The ring of muscle in his oesophagus which should stop vomit surging back up into the mouth was exceptionally weak. Despite multiple medications, everything dripped down his feeding tube came back up, and once, he aspirated the vomit – breathed it back in – giving him a lung infection which could have been deadly. For a time he was fed through a tube into his intestines, to bypass his unhappy stomach, but the body is not designed to absorb nutrients that way and a long-term solution had to be found. The only possibility, the doctors explained, was surgery.

In an elegant, fairly major operation called a Nissen's fundoplication,[†] the top of the stomach (the fundus) is wrapped completely around the lower part of the oesophagus to reinforce the weak muscle, so stomach contents can't easily slip back up the oesophagus. These days, a Nissen's is usually done with minimally invasive keyhole surgery. The surgeon makes a few small cuts in the abdomen, into which tiny instruments are inserted. They also insert, into the tummy button, a laparoscope – a telescopic tube with a camera and light attached, which sends back magnified video images to a monitor the surgeon watches as the operation is performed. Carbon dioxide gas is pumped into the abdomen to inflate it, so the surgeon has a clear view and plenty of room. The operation had various risks, from the scary-sounding 'dumping syndrome' in which food travels too fast through the stomach, causing diarrhoea and retching, to swallowing problems. Joel's stomach would be made smaller, and he might never be able to burp or vomit again. But, at risk of aspirating vomit, this was the only answer for him.

There would be another element to the surgery, too. Because of the reflux, it had not been safe to wean Joel off tube feeds into his intestines and try breastfeeding. Even once he could safely use his oesophagus and stomach as a result of the fundoplication, it would take time to gain the ability to feed through his mouth, because, having now been tube-fed for three months, he had lost the instinct. To him, a mouth was

† This eponymous operation was developed in the 1950s by Rudolph Nissen, a Jewish surgeon who escaped Nazi Germany and famously performed abdominal surgery on Albert Einstein. Afterwards, Einstein was photographed sticking out his tongue at press photographers. He sent a clipping of the iconic photograph to Nissen with the note: 'To Nissen my tummy / The world my tongue'.

not associated with food – but instead with tubes being pushed down it.

So, after the fundoplication, the surgeon would do a gastrostomy. A small hole in the wall of the stomach would be opened up, and a 'button' inserted which looks like the plug on a paddling pool. It would be held in place by a balloon filled with water beneath the stomach wall. Having flipped up the cap of this button, we would need to attach a tube with a key at the end. The key, turned in one direction, would open the passage to the stomach. The other end of the tube would attach to a plungerless syringe, into which we would pour milk. It would flow into the tube, and through the button, directly into Joel's stomach. This way, he could be fed, and at the same time, we would try to teach him to drink (and, when he was old enough, eat) using his mouth. Only when he could eat enough orally to sustain himself could the button be removed, at which point the wound in the stomach should heal naturally. It might take years for Joel to eat orally. He might be a teenager.

By the time of his operation, Joel had been in the neonatal unit for three months. The day before the operation, the 'transport' came to take him the short distance across Bloomsbury to Great Ormond Street Hospital (GOSH). Joel was locked into an incubator on wheels and rolled away onto an ambulance, packaged like a lab specimen kept under glass, or a monkey being sent out to space in a space capsule. In that coffin-like pod, he had never seemed so unreachable.

I walked the twenty minutes to the hospital, and found my way to the general surgery ward, Squirrel. At the time, it was temporarily housed in an old and rather decrepit part of the hospital, with gloomy, narrow corridors. I was shown to a small room with a single bed for me, and a large blue-barred cot for

Joel. I felt very worried about this. Didn't the people at GOSH know that Joel slept in an incubator, and was nursed in an open high dependency ward? He had never been left 'alone' in a room. Here, although Joel had a nurse, she wasn't constantly in the room with him. But I was assured he would be carefully monitored; the nurses would check on him through the night.

I had become so used to 'our' hospital that GOSH's seemingly more relaxed approach was a culture shock. Here, in a general surgery ward rather than a neonatal unit, I quickly observed, there was no yellow line, no absolute insistence on hand washing on entering any space. I watched in horror as a doctor dropped a pen on the floor, picked it up and carried on as normal. I would have run the pen and my hands under the hot tap with soap, dried them with paper towels, and coated them in sanitizing gel.

I had never been able to lie down in the same place as Joel. Never been able to sit on a bed, with him lying next to me. Never been able to walk out of a doorway into another room holding him. Now I was free to do all this.

That night I couldn't decide whether to be happy to spend time 'alone' with Joel, or to let myself sleep at all. But by morning, I had learned something about him. I knew he didn't lie awake crying in the early hours. And I had been able to look after him, in my own way – mainly, calling the nurse every time the sleep apnoea mat Joel slept on alarmed (each time, the alarm was false). Still, I wanted Joel to go onto the open part of the ward where he would be more visible to the nurses, and I was relieved when he was moved.

Luckily, Joel was first on the list for surgery that morning. He didn't have to be 'starved' too long. We were not always so fortunate and I was later to learn how having to distract your child from their hunger for hour upon hour in the morning of surgery is a torture of its own.

The surgeon was Kate Cross, a cool blonde businesslike Australian only four years older than me and also (I only learned as a journalist, when Joel was no longer her patient) a mother, whose two children were not much older than Joel. Kate starts work early in the morning and, if not on call, is home by nine at night, when her children are already in bed. Later, she told me how she used to meet her husband in a park near the hospital. He would bring her baby for her to feed, and she would hand over expressed milk. At the time of Joel's surgery, though, she seemed so mighty and impressive that I thought of her more as some kind of superhuman, and Phil and I assumed she could not be a mother.

It was only when I wrote this book that we would meet again. Then, Kate Cross told me how, growing up in the New South Wales countryside, just north of Sydney, her brother was unwell and spent a lot of time in hospital. There were times when the family thought he was going to die.

The young Kate spent a lot of time watching people caring for him. This was when she decided she wanted to be a children's doctor. Then, doing her medical training, she fell in love with surgery – a field where a doctor can make a big, concrete difference. Operating on an infant is not just about cutting and sewing in miniature. Babies' bodies work differently from adults and older children – they breathe faster; their hearts beat quicker; more of their body weight is water so they can dehydrate easily; the kidneys and liver are not yet working at mature strength. Premature babies are even weaker, unable to control their body temperature or breathe or swallow, their veins as thin as spiderwebs. As the American paediatric surgeon Catherine Musemeche wrote in her memoir *Small*, 'Their organs are like Jell-O and barely hold together when our imposing adult fingers push and pull.'[2]

'There's no margin for error, so everything you have to do has to be very delicate and very precise,' Kate Cross told me of neonatal surgery, 'and that's one of the joys, because you are able to really hone your skills and be as delicate and precise, and it's lovely surgery. It really is lovely.'

'What do you mean, lovely?' I asked, surprised by her choice of word.

'There is an art to surgery,' she replied. 'We're really drawing parallels between what we do from a surgical perspective and a musician who makes beautiful music with their hands.' She enters a heightened state of awareness – 'a real sense of clarity' – while operating, like an athlete preparing for a race, or a performer about to go on stage.

I asked to look at her hands. Was there something magical about them? Nothing that I could see, though Kate flashed me her broad smile: 'If I drink too much coffee, they shake . . . if I know that I'm doing very fine surgery I won't have too much coffee.'

I asked if she remembered operating on Joel. Yes, she said. 'The reason I remember Joel's operation is because we were worried he was small and he had the cardiac side of things.'

She had seemed achingly confident to me, but she told me she was always conscious of her own fallibility. 'You do get nervous,' she said. 'I think you *need* to get nervous to some extent. The last thing you want is a surgeon who's so confident and relaxed they lose some of that edge.'

Children's surgeons have to shut off their natural human responses and separate the technical task from the fact they are holding the life of a little boy or girl in their hands, or they would become daunted. 'You don't forget that they're a little baby, but you can't have that emotional feeling,' Kate told me – if she saw me in the park, she said, it would be a different interaction from when she is in her professional role. 'You can't think about the child in the same way you would if you were a mum, because actually I'm there with a job to do.'

That day in 2011, my baby facing surgery, I was the anxious mother, and Miss Cross was the brisk professional. Our interactions were quite limited; being a surgeon, she was incredibly busy, and Phil and I were used to waiting hours for a ten minute Q&A with her. I saw her registrars and senior house officers, and the nurses, jump to Miss Cross's every command. I felt admiration bordering on a crush. This was to be one of the hardest times for Joel. My baby was in good hands with Miss Cross, I felt.

The list of possible (though highly unlikely) risks, including death, was read out to us. Miss Cross had often described Joel's 'tummy', including us as parents in the simple and safe-sounding nursery language, but now I saw the stark scribble in the doctor's hand of what they were going to do to bodily organs, under my son's name, which I had to consent to and sign. I dressed Joel for his operation in his froggy suit – a sleep-suit shaped like a sleeping bag. I tried to think of Miss Cross, how she could get him out easily as it had a flap at the bottom.

It was just another day, for Joel. Unsuspecting, he was wheeled through the hospital to the theatre floor. Carried by adrenaline, I was still amazed at just being able to walk beside him, anywhere. We were shown into the little anaesthetic room. The anaesthetist was kind, so kind I knew this was going to be bad. Joel lay on my lap. The mask with its fearful artificial smell came near. The moment had come. His body stiffened in panic. He tried to escape the smell. He could not.

We were betraying him. But he also needed us and I felt him wordlessly begging us to save him from this. And we could not, would not. His eyes rolled blank, and I placed him on the bed, stole a last kiss, and walked away, leaving him alone.

Four hours later, as we waited on the ward, the call came. All had gone well. We could go and see Joel in recovery.

There he was, lying on a bed in a small row of children waking from operations. A nurse was standing over him, watching him very closely. Here was my boy again, still intact, asleep. What had he undergone? On his once-smooth belly now were small, neat cuts where the instruments for keyhole surgery had gone in, twisting and turning. The froggy suit was folded neatly next to him at the bottom of the bed. Imagining someone taking off that froggy suit made me feel especially sad. That person had found the little flap at the bottom of the sleepsuit and eased out the body I had so carefully hidden. The sleepsuit was just a folly. Joel had been stripped of something in having an operation, not just his clothes but any normality they signified.

His eyes were open and afraid, full of tears, and he writhed. 'He's in pain,' I said, my tears streaming. The nurse, full of compassion, was already giving a dose of morphine. Joel's eyes rolled back, and he fell mercifully unconscious again. The nurse seemed far more concerned about me than Joel and asked if I needed to sit down.

Every time Joel returned to consciousness, he returned to pain. And was sent back to sleep every twenty minutes on a tide of morphine.

He was wheeled to the ward; I crouched over his trolley all the way, stroking his forehead and arms. Phil and I, our parents, our sisters and my friend Grace kept a twenty-four-hour vigil at Joel's cot, taking turns to sit on the bedside chair, and gradually the pain became less. Then, in the middle of one night, he suddenly went white and struggled to breathe. My sister shouted and ran for a doctor, but Grace – cheerful and from the outside world – calmly said to me: 'Look, his chest's going up and down.' Joel had developed pulmonary oedema – fluid in the lungs. A young, harassed-looking doctor administered a diuretic, and Joel's colour returned.

It was a relief the next evening when a nurse taking over night duty told us he wouldn't leave Joel's side. He propped Joel upwards and showed us how to hold the oxygen mask so he could breathe more easily, and efficiently sorted out Joel's notes and nursing station. 'If this is in chaos, it's no good, is it?' he tutted. He chatted to Joel like a buddy, boy to boy, and we sensed Joel's contentment. That young nurse has always stayed in my family's minds.

I will also never forget the family whose daughter, Zoe, was in the cot next to Joel's at GOSH. She was a few years old and had spent many months there; in fact she had spent much of her life in hospital, her parents spending every day there with her. With complex health problems, she had slipped down the rabbit hole, into a hospital life where no end was in sight.

A few days after Joel's operation, now fed through the gastrostomy and no longer vomiting, Joel was sent safely back to his incubator at UCH. Phil and I have often thought about young Zoe, though, who seemed to have little hope of leaving the ward at GOSH. A couple of years after Joel came home, on an outpatient visit, we bumped into the family, still there.

*

Joel went on to have three more operations at Great Ormond Street as a young child – two more minor ones on his stomach, at ages two and three, when he had started to eat and drink and the gastrostomy button had been taken out, but the wound failed to heal on its own; and one more major one aged four – open heart surgery to fix a hole in the atrial septum, the barrier between the two upper chambers – atria – of the heart.

Atrial septal defects (ASDs) are the commonest congenital heart malformation. An ASD allows blood to pass from the left to the right atrium, and when an ASD is large, like Joel's, the right side of the heart becomes overloaded with blood. Fixing a hole in the heart, ideally done just before a child starts school, when they are big but the operation won't impact their education, is the bread and butter of congenital cardiac surgery. It's so low-key for surgeons today that it's hard to remember that only a couple of generations ago, before modern heart surgery, a large ASD, like other congenital heart conditions, was a death sentence. It would eventually cause deterioration of the heart and lungs in middle age and an early death – and before the ultrasound era, an ASD's very existence might well have gone unnoticed until symptoms arose.

But these days, a child predisposed to a heart condition because of having a syndrome like Noonan's, or who has a murmur a doctor can hear with a stethoscope, is given a simple heart echo scan, and a problem like an ASD shows up clearly. (In the pre-ultrasound age, a heart murmur, caused by the sound of blood pouring through a hole in the heart, was often as far as diagnosis could go for heart trouble – a vague label for something wrong.) Usually an ASD is fixed using a minimally invasive procedure. Under general anaesthetic, a long thin tube – a catheter – is pushed into a vein at the top of the child's leg and towards the heart. A device rather like a closed umbrella is pushed through the catheter and once it reaches the hole in the heart, the umbrella is opened and the hole is closed. Finally the catheter is pulled out.

But in Joel's case, there wasn't just one hole. His atrial septum was punched with multiple holes, like Swiss cheese. And there wasn't enough of a ridge in his heart on which to prop open the umbrella device. Because of the particular structure of his heart, it had to be fixed with open heart surgery – cutting the chest open, stopping the heart while maintaining circulation on a bypass machine, and sewing the hole-filled septum shut – still a ridiculously basic operation for a heart surgeon, but, of course, anything but basic for us.

I learned a few things from my son having an operation every year of his life until the age of four.

One is that the thought of open heart surgery makes people gasp – a heart condition strikes us as the most fundamental health problem of all, it seems – but in fact, Joel's recovery from his stomach surgery seemed more painful, because of all the muscles in the abdomen.

Another is that cardiac intensive care is a quiet place, rather than full of shouting and panic as I had always imagined. I was used to the subtropically heated rooms and myriad bleating machines of neonatal intensive care, but the cardiac intensive care ward at Great Ormond Street was airy and oddly peaceful. I soon realized it was because all the children were on life support and couldn't breathe for themselves. They were all unconscious or semi-conscious, and heavily sedated with morphine.

That's another thing I learned about – morphine. Specifically, what it's like to see your child's eyes roll back into oblivion when the morphine dose kicks in. The fact is, they look like a drug addict in the body of a baby. It seems unnatural. And yet when the morphine wears off, you're the one pressing the button on the driver to give them the next dose the second it's available.

The high dependency ward is, maybe, harder than intensive care. A child is moved there once they are breathing in air on their own, perhaps with the help of a little oxygen mask or nasal prongs. Here, often, complications emerge in the middle of the night: strange heart rhythms; pulmonary oedema. In high dependency, a child wakes fully from surgery and the morphine is scaled back rapidly, replaced by plain paracetamol and ibuprofen. It's here that the pain takes over from the post-operative daze, and here that they start fighting all the drains and wires attached to their body. Joel was only in a room with a bed for Phil or me beside his when he was essentially out of danger; when he was in the intensive care and high dependency wards after surgery, we sat beside him on a chair all night. Singing helped the long hours pass, I found: for some reason I often sang Joel 'Morning Has Broken'. Actors came to the ward we were in once, but none of the children was well enough to watch them and instead they played to visiting siblings.

Those nights in intensive care and high dependency at GOSH, I was allocated a room shared with another mother in the 'nurses' home' at the back of the hospital. When Phil took his turn at Joel's bedside, I would walk there at 4 a.m. to get some sleep, down silent corridors empty but for the occasional other wild-haired, grey-faced parent. Having found my room, I had to make up a single bed with sticky plastic duvets and pillows, and I lay awake, wired, listening to the other mother's steady breathing. I would rise after four hours of fruitless tossing and turning, shower in an institutional bathroom block, then hurry back to Joel.

Despite not being religious, at times like these I found myself seeking out places of prayer. I felt safe in churches, where the whole and only point was to wish for good, but often I found them locked. At GOSH, my sister and I went on a quest to find the hospital chapel. It was tucked away on a basement floor, past a hydrotherapy pool. The small room was filled with photographs of children who had died and tributes to them. We sat and prayed silently.

Over Joel's four operations, all of which went smoothly, I repeatedly found the same two moments the most difficult. First was what happened in the anaesthetic room. The forced jollity as Phil and I faked smiles and upbeat voices to keep Joel calm as we carried him down the corridors towards it (later he rode there on Phil's shoulders and another time, blithely on a red toy motorcycle), his tiny unsuspecting body shielded only by a thin, brightly coloured hospital gown, a lamb to the slaughter.

By the time Joel was four, he was so averse to doctors and hospitals that, with the help of a specialist cardiac psychologist and two play specialists, we prepared him for surgery in a very particular way. First, we spent weeks playing with doctors' kits and reading books about going to hospital, the body and in particular the heart. Joel was visited weekly at home by a play therapist who brought real medical equipment like oxygen masks, stethoscopes and cannulas for him to examine, as well as bags of toy ambulances and hospitals. Next, we told him that his heart wasn't working perfectly and needed to be fixed, using the analogy of an engine which needs to go to the garage. Then, we visited Great Ormond Street, just to play and look around. Finally, about four days before the surgery, we broke the news that he was going to have the operation to fix his heart and told him a bit more about it – going for a 'special sleep', and the fact it might hurt when he woke (I have always felt it essential to be honest so that Joel knows he can trust us). All this planning, and the fact Joel didn't know what was about to happen for a long time, made it hard not to cry whenever I talked about the surgery. I dreaded having to be strong for him because I was the person he needed the most.

Our preparations helped, but, as I was to learn fully only years later, Joel was too young to understand, and it was his lack of understanding which seemed the worst betrayal of his trust in us, his protectors. It was like seeing a defenceless animal suffer; you cannot explain to an animal that the vet is helping it, not attacking it. We would enter the little anaesthetic room through one door and see the double doors opposite that our son would go through next, the assembly line leading to the operating theatre. The kind – always kind – anaesthetist would immediately take control. There would be bubbles blown by a nurse, jokes, anything we could think of to distract Joel as he sat on my lap cuddling me and piping up: 'I don't like this room.' In later years, they had already given him a pre-med tranquillizer to calm him. It made no difference. As soon as the plastic mask came close to him, hissing its alien, unnatural fluorescent pen smell, Joel instinctively recoiled. I could under-stand his fear – I had never had an anaesthetic myself, but I also found the insistent, harsh smell of the gas somehow petri-fying. 'I don't like it,' Joel would say, twisting to escape the mask, his voice rising. 'I DON'T LIKE IT. MUMMY, SCARED.' I couldn't help him. The only way to help him was not to save him from this monster. There was no calm count-ing from ten to one. Just his desperate fight as the anaesthetist held the mask near his face and he struggled until his eyes rolled back, still open, and with a sudden guttural snore, his body succumbed, helplessly, to unconsciousness.

'Quick as you like, put him on the bed,' the anaesthetist would say, gently but firmly. 'Give him a kiss, we'll take care of him, we promise.' Joel's apparently lifeless body would be lifted onto a gurney, and I would turn back to take one last look, take in the bustle already beginning around him. The door would swing closed behind us and, awkwardly trying to hide my emotion, I'd be hugged by a nurse, and led away, to wait for news.

The second dreadful moment was when Joel regained consciousness. It was not just the sight of his little body multilated by strange drains and tubes. It was the fact he was too young to understand why he was in pain. Every time he came around, he whimpered in shock. I could feel his thought: 'Where am I?' As I leaned in to kiss him, I would breathe in the anaesthetic fug rolling off his tongue, his body filled with it, radiating it.

After the heart surgery, Joel woke up in intensive care on a ventilator. The only mark on his chest was a surprisingly neat narrow plaster, but he had a chest drain, and various other wires attached to him. In the words of children's cardiac surgeon Kate Bull, 'There is something appalling about seeing a tube coming out of your chest and dropping red stuff into a jar on the floor . . . the visceral revulsion of seeing bloody pipes coming out of a child's body does not come from a rational place.'[3] Joel started trying to turn from lying on his back and tugging at the tube in his throat. Suddenly, an alarm sounded.

It was only when I saw a crash team of doctors and nurses sprinting to Joel, with a defibrillator ready to shock his heart, that I realized the alarm was for him. To make way for the doctors I backed out of the room, shaking, an equally confused junior nurse putting her arm around me. What was happening? All I could see was a crowd of doctors holding a doll-small boy upright over his bed.

Minutes later the emergency was over, the doctors smiling and strolling away while my family stood, aghast. Eventually, a nurse explained it to us. Joel had managed to pull the ventilator out of his throat; it had got stuck halfway. He had stopped breathing and his oxygen level had dropped, leaving him blue. Now the doctors had got it out, and he was breathing well with a little oxygen mask on the sheet beside him.

For adults, open heart surgery is massive. After a bad night in high dependency, Joel bounced back from major surgery as only a child can. His operation was on a Wednesday. By Saturday, he was in his pyjamas pedalling a tricycle in the hospital play centre, and that evening he was home. In his frailty for the next few weeks I got another glimpse of him as an old man rather than a child, yet his abiding memory of this last operation is, thankfully, not of pain but of riding the red motorbike.

Not long after Joel left hospital, I started an anonymous blog about mothering a sick baby. Helen, a kind, bookish mother of two, came across my blog and started liking my posts. Soon, we met up in the real world; we lived close by. Helen's children were healthy, but she was always curious and supportive about my world of tube-feeding and developmental delay. Years later, while I was writing this book, Helen had a third child, who seemed well until in a routine afterbirth check, a heart murmur was found, and now it was my turn to be supportive.

Helen's baby Gilly had severe tetralogy of Fallot (pronounced fallow), a congenital defect caused by a combination of four (*tetra* in Greek) structural abnormalities in the heart. Blood picks up oxygen as it circulates through the lungs. Moved along by the pumping heart, blood delivers this rich red oxygen to every cell in the body, where it's unloaded and used as energy. Then, the de-oxygenated blood – now a purple-blue colour – returns to the heart, where it's sent back to the lungs on another circuit. A lot of congenital heart problems involve faults in the circuit so that blue blood ends up where it shouldn't, causing a cascade of problems. Tetralogy of Fallot's nickname is 'blue baby syndrome'. The pulmonary artery (the blood vessel that carries blood to pick up oxygen in the lungs) is narrowed, which thickens the right ventricle (the heart's right pumping chamber), causing a blockage. This combines with a ventricular septal defect (VSD), a particularly troublesome kind of hole in the heart, in this case worsened by occurring right next to the aorta, the body's largest blood vessel. De-oxygenated blood crosses through the VSD into the left ventricle and gets into the aorta, which should instead channel oxygen-rich blood. A baby's crying or constipation can set off a 'blue spell' in which the baby is deprived of oxygen and needs to be rushed to hospital.

Until the moment of placing three-month-old Gilly in the anaesthetist's arms, Helen was responsible for her child. Then the doors slammed and Helen and her husband joined the other crying parents in the corridor. To fill the time they had breakfast and Helen – a phlegmatic civil servant – had a haircut, pretending to be a normal person having a day out in London. One can imagine the awkward conversation with the hairdresser asking, 'Doing anything special today?' and Helen muttering, 'No, not really.' Like when someone dies and you feel you should spend hours crying but can't, when your child is having major surgery, there is only so much time you can spend wringing your hands. Helen's story reminded me of how during Joel's open heart surgery, I distracted myself by watching *Homes Under the Hammer*, a lightweight daytime TV show about people doing up auctioned properties.

Bizarrely, because I focused so intently on it as a distraction and it took my mind to a safe place, it was one of the most enjoyable episodes of daytime TV I have ever seen.

Seeing Gilly in intensive care, her face swollen and wires coming out of her, that strange anaesthetic smell on her breath, all Helen could do was kiss her and stroke her hair. On the second day after surgery, Gilly developed chylothorax – during surgery one of her lymph vessels had been nicked and now it was leaking into her chest. But it was only when the doctors explained that now Gilly would need a special diet and could no longer be fed expressed milk that Helen found herself unable to stop crying. In her working life, Helen plays a senior role. Now, she found it 'weird to be so disempowered', listening to ward rounds which she didn't understand. Complications followed. Gilly could not be weaned from the ventilator. Then she got fluid in her lungs and around her heart. Helen, staying in the nurses' home as I had and still hardly able to hold Gilly, wanted to be told 'everything's going to be fine' but no one could reassure her. She believed Gilly was going to die.

Gilly reached high dependency, but there, miserable on CPAP, she struggled to breathe. Helen became depressed, consumed with fears of death and missing her other children. Finally, after nearly a month, Gilly was well enough to go home, but there she wouldn't drink her formula. They were soon back in their local hospital. In the wards on the weekend, it was so lonely that Helen rang the Samaritans. There was nothing much they could say to help, though.

Gilly's life was saved, but before the era of modern surgery – and outside the developed world where such surgery is affordable and takes place – a person with tetralogy of Fallot gradually becomes more and more starved of oxygen, until all the body's organs are damaged. If the baby had the extraordinary luck to survive childhood, they would still almost certainly die by middle age.[4] Gilly shouldn't need another heart operation until at least her twenties and can expect a long, active life,[5] but she will always need to be under a cardiologist's care. Speaking a few months after the surgery, cuddling a grizzling Gilly, Helen told me she found the experience terrifying and that she felt her bond with her baby had been damaged in a way she found hard to explain. A year on, that bond had recovered, but Helen still had to work hard not to think about the surgery too much. Her consciousness of life's fragility has been permanently altered.

*

As fetal and neonatal medicine were taking off, surgeons were also daring to raise the apparently crazy question: could they repair a congenitally diseased heart (or other organ) at birth or soon after?[6]

The idea of doing surgery on a baby was not exactly new. Babies have been circumcised since ancient times. In eleventh-century Spain, the Spanish-Arabic doctor Albucasis described cauterizing the skin and draining fluid from infants born with hydrocephalus (fluid in the brain) and opening a newborn's obstructed urinary tract,[7] and in the late 1600s, the Swiss surgeon Johannes Fatio operated on infants with exomphalos and, remarkably, even successfully separated conjoined twins, a feat not to be repeated until the twentieth century.[8] But back then, operating on anyone, especially babies, was agonizing and quite likely to be deadly. A baby with a serious birth defect was almost certainly doomed. Only in the mid-nineteenth century, with anaesthesia and antisepsis bringing the possibility of safely fixing congenital defects, did children's hospitals like CHOP and GOSH spring up.

Yet it took until the 1940s for operating on children to get off the ground as a specialty – at Boston Children's Hospital and CHOP, helped by the first antibiotics. Even then the mortality rate was prohibitively high. There were no such things as intensive care ventilators or IV catheters yet. And anaesthesia was so dangerous for children's small bodies that surgeons feared using it in case a child never woke again.[9] Other doctors widely viewed paediatric surgeons with scorn, believing children were just scaled-down adults and their surgeons needed no special training.[10]

But then one of the first paediatric surgeons – Charles Everett Koop, who set up the children's surgery department at CHOP and later became the US Surgeon General – worked out with his anaesthetist colleague Margo Deming how to anaesthetize children safely, by pumping carefully regulated amounts of anaesthetic through a tube into the windpipe. This technique is a staple of anaesthesia today, but back then, before plastic tubing and monitors, Koop and Deming had to make their own equipment from rubber and then, after the operations, sat up all night watching over their patients. Koop also realized that children were not miniature adults; they required their own special treatments. For example, an essentially healthy child doesn't need much bed rest after an operation (after Joel's heart surgery, the nurses made him get up and walk within forty-eight hours).

A Christian convert, Koop, like other early pioneers of fetal and neonatal medicine, was ardently against abortion ('my concern about the *un*born followed as the night the day my concern about the *newly* born,' he wrote).[11] He felt hugely for sick babies and their parents – not only human ones. One day his resident started to tell him rather hesitantly about a new-born with intestinal obstruction. After giving a complete history, the resident said: 'The only thing unusual about this patient is – it's an orang-utan.' The baby orang-utan from Philadelphia zoo had been kept alive so far by a young vet who took her home and nursed her in her own bed with a baby bottle. Koop agreed to operate, and the baby grew up. 'When I last heard, she was being courted by a young male orang-utan at Memphis zoo,' Koop later recalled.

The highlight of his surgical career was taking on a seem-ingly impossible case of fourteen-month-old conjoined twins from the Dominican Republic called Clara and Alta Rod-ríguez. The girls shared a colon and liver, had four vaginas, and their urinary tracts were entwined. The parents were told they could not be separated, but the twins' aunt was a maid for a Philadelphia woman, who asked Koop for help. He got them to Philadelphia and did everything for free. When conjoined, the girls were driving each other mad, punching and scratch-ing but unable to get away from each other. After the successful separation surgery, one reached out to touch her sister's hand across the bedsheet.

Sadly, two years later, Alta, sitting on the porch of her home, popped a bean into her mouth which became lodged in her vocal cords – which ironically would have been harder to treat than the complex surgery she had endured. She choked to death.

Losses stayed with Koop always, and he cherished his bonds with parents who had been through devastating loss, in some cases becoming close friends. Haunted in the 1960s by an idea that he was becoming almost too good at comforting grieving parents, Koop had a disturbing premonition that he would lose one of his own children. Then, tragically, in 1968, his son David was killed while mountain climbing. After that, Koop could 'rarely discuss the death of a child without tears welling up'.

If surgery is hard for families today, it used to be ten times worse. Children's heart surgery happened for almost twenty years before anyone thought about preparing children (or parents) emotionally.[12] The few children who had heart surgery before the 1980s usually had to stay on adult wards and were separated from their parents.[13] In the 1960s it was customary for children on IVs to be restrained, ankles and arms tied to the bedrails, and for babies to be wedged into an unmovable position with sandbags.[14]

Although Britain's first surgical unit for neonates was set up in 1953 at the Alder Hey Children's Hospital in Liverpool, it wasn't until the 1980s that neonatal and paediatric intensive care specialists and units became common in hospitals, using the recently invented ventilators and CPAP and sustaining babies on TPN, nutrition delivered through their veins. Once doctors learned to interpret the 'snowstorm' pictures of early ultrasound echoes and accurately pinpoint the mysteries of a sick infant's body, surgery became an increasingly safe option. But even in the early 1980s, there were still no intensive care doctors at Great Ormond Street, so it was up to the surgeons to look after children after operations – with far less sophisticated drugs and monitors than today.[15]

Still, the invention of the heart-lung machine in the 1950s and the discovery in the 1970s of a life-saving hormone drug called prostaglandin opened the door for neonatal cardiac surgery. Prostaglandin keeps a blood vessel called the ductus arteriosus open so that blood keeps moving, even if there is a life-threatening obstruction elsewhere in the heart. This bought cardiac surgeons more crucial time – instead of having

to operate immediately and do dangerous things to unbelievably sick children in a rush, they could wait a few hours or
days for the child's metabolism to stabilize thanks to the hormone, and work in far more stable conditions. By the late
1980s, GOSH was doing heart transplants for children.[16]

Compared to adult cardiac surgery – a limited repertoire
of mending coronary arteries, valves and aortas – there is a
multitude of congenital heart problems which send children
to the operating theatre. In the early days, neonatal heart surgery attracted risk-takers willing to take on the cases no one
else was prepared to do, who enjoyed the danger much as
some people like motor-racing. The Florida surgeon Tom
Karl once said: 'surgery is like a narcotic', and Luca Vricella
from Johns Hopkins University: 'If I have to describe the
feeling of operating on a newborn heart . . . the perfect analogy is that of driving a car at 200 mph on a single lane with
water on either side . . . I think it's the most exhilarating, yet
humbling, experience that you can possibly have.' Oliver
Ghez of the Royal Brompton Hospital has recalled the first
time he operated on a newborn and how 'I really realized
how mad you have to be to do this.' For Tom Karl, 'the first
time I was involved in a newborn operation it was like a religious experience . . . I couldn't believe what we were doing . . .
I was really just taken to another place.'[17]

*

As a mother, the two worst moments – immediately before
and after each operation – were the gates to a time and place
in my child's life I had no access to, perhaps the most dangerous

moments and places of his life, when he was on an operating table, in the hands of strangers, far from the 'real' world.

I still didn't know exactly what had happened after I left Joel in the anaesthetic room, and before he was given back to me, covered in tubing. So to find out what happens in this world unknown by the public and even by parents, I went back to Great Ormond Street to observe.

The journey was familiar: the long queue to go up in the lifts at Russell Square Tube; gradually exchanging streams of office workers for children in wheelchairs as you near the hospital. The drab hotels, one with an emblem of a ship on its front. The wound-up feeling inside. The unsparing greyness of the streets.

At 8 a.m., I took the lift up to the operating theatres and was buzzed through. I was to watch Joel's heart surgeon, Martin Kostolny, operate on a little girl. If doctors are the gods of our times, the power of life and death in their hands, then surgeons are the gods' gods, and surgeons who operate on small children the gods' gods' gods, and those children's surgeons who work on hearts are seen as deities almost beyond measure. I had very few memories of Mr Kostolny – a middle-aged man who spoke in a quiet, precise way – from Joel's operation. In fact we had only met him briefly on the morning of surgery and seen him a second and last time when he checked on Joel afterwards. All the other discussions had been with his team, mainly his registrar. And of course, though very polite, Mr Kostolny now told me in his understated way that he had no memory of Joel at all. For him it had been an utterly insignificant case – an ASD repair being the simplest kind of open heart surgery, and everything having gone just as it should.

A motherly nurse called Maureen showed me the locker room where I had to change into scrubs. It took me ten minutes to find a blue T-shirt and trousers that were neither too big nor too small from the unlabelled mountain of clothes. I also had to borrow purple plastic shoes with Mickey Mouse buttons on, a paper cap to cover my hair and a mask to go over my nose and mouth, which felt suffocating even when tied loose. I wondered at the staff all around me who wore their masks neat and tight, and managed to breathe. Looking like one of them, I had crossed over. I felt the anonymity of the mask, through which all emotions were hidden, and the androgynous uniform of the scrubs we all wore – in this costume, we became nearly robotic, and feelings seemed less important. It had started snowing a blizzard outside, but all medical staff were present. In the NHS there is no option of a snow day.

I entered the anaesthetic room a few minutes after the parents of the three-year-old girl had left, the mother crying in a nurse's arms. An anaesthetist's role is to keep the child stable while lots of other people do harmful things. Some say they are more risk-averse than surgeons. The classic description is that their work is 99 per cent boredom and 1 per cent blind panic – though of course the best anaesthetists are the ones who stay calm in a panic situation.

Despite a pre-med, the girl had been very anxious – understandably, since this was to be her fourth heart operation – and had had a 'total meltdown' before falling unconscious, the consultant anaesthetist Ellen (as she introduced herself to me) told me. I recognized her as one of Joel's anaesthetists – blonde and thin, wearing trainers, brisk yet friendly and unpretentious in a very British way, and, as such, infinitely reassuring. This was a safe pair of hands.

The operation was a 'redo'. The girl had a complex cardiac history. She had had two heart operations before – an atrioventricular septal defect (a double hole in the centre of the heart, also affecting the valves between the top and bottom heart chambers) was repaired, but unfortunately she had come back with severe subaortic stenosis: narrowing where the blood leaves the left side of the heart. That was repaired, but now something was wrong again. The doctors thought she was developing narrowing again – today, the aim was to find and remove the blockage. The heart's slow beat had also been causing alarm since the second heart operation. At times the child had been in complete heart block – a serious condition when the electrical impulses which control heartbeats fail to pass between the top and bottom chambers of the heart, and the heart's rhythm breaks down. Now they were going to implant a pacemaker. On top of this, the stomach was malrotated – the spleen and stomach were in a rather strange position, which would complicate today's operation.

I had wondered if I'd find it hard to watch an operation. But I didn't. The only moments I felt tearful were the same as the moments I'd found difficult as a parent – the before and the after, when a child is still obviously a child. For the surgery in the middle, I learned that childishness, unconscious and covered up in drapes, is somehow less obvious. It is perhaps the anaesthetist, the gatekeeper who guides the child across the bridge between the safe 'real' world and the dangerous world of surgery and back, who is closest to the child and the family, rather than the surgeon.

When a child resists anaesthesia, as this girl and my own son did, Ellen told me later, 'It's ghastly. If I have a bad induction, I feel I've completely failed.' Some children, she said, love the smell of the sleepy gas, but even then, it goes against a parent's instincts 'to see them go floppy and leave them with strangers'. She often uses nitrous oxide – laughing gas, the 'gas and air' used in childbirth – which doesn't smell, to start the anaesthesia; it gets the child two-thirds of the way to sleep. I asked Ellen if she herself had ever had an operation. She had, she said, and she feared dying during it very much. It can happen. This is why every parent whose child is about to have surgery has to be warned explicitly, with the utmost delicacy, that there is a small chance their child could die. Ellen has, in her working life, seen patients die in theatre – usually older people, but, also, incredibly rarely, a child. Usually when a child dies in surgery, she told me, the writing has been on the wall; the surgery an obviously risky last resort for a child whose body is failing. What is really rare, she said, is when you don't expect a death. 'Those are the cases written on your soul,' she said.

Now, as I saw the child for the first time, her fine blonde hair French-plaited in pigtails, lying freshly anaesthetized and ventilated on a puffy paper blanket on the gurney, I felt a jolt. The doors to Theatre 7 were now open. She slept with her eyes slightly open, as Joel had done. Soon her eyelids were taped down. Her hospital gown covered in balloons was pulled down – exposing a chest already scarred from her previous heart operations – and finally removed and folded away, replaced by paper sheets. Her face was covered by thin transparent plastic like a sweetie wrapper and they scrubbed her skin with 'fake tan', an orange antiseptic. Lines were placed and finally her back was arched over a small bolster so her chest pointed up. At 9.30 a.m., she was wheeled into theatre.

The large room was soon filled with people, trolleys, machines and lights. The child was laid out and her nakedness covered in layers of paper and plastic and cotton wool, then blue drapes. I had never seen a body look so vulnerable. Her face was behind the drapes – all the surgeons could see of her, in the end, was a small orange painted area of her chest where they were cutting. With her once scared, now sleeping face hidden to all but the anaesthetists, she became an anonymous and unnatural-coloured piece of flesh and there was no call for emotion.

At the back of the room, two surgeons scrubbed up in a long sink and had their gowns tied back. A camera over the child's chest would broadcast their work on TV screens which magnify the view a hundred times to be visible to everyone else in the room. A child's heart is the size of their fist – this girl's, then, the size of a clementine. The star of the show, Martin Kostolny, would only arrive later to do the most complex part of the operation: to cut through the aorta, go through the aortic valve and look into the left ventricle and remove the cause of the blockage.

Stacks of scissors were lined up. In the corner, a digital clock was started. The heart-lung machine I sat behind was a spaghetti junction of red-filled tubes. At 10 a.m., the first cut was made and by 10.15 the heart was visible, pulsating in the cranked-open chest. Now the surgeons began scraping painstakingly through gossamer layers of tissue.

Martin Kostolny unobtrusively entered the room at 10.30, just as the other surgeons fully exposed the pinkish-white heart, flecked with blood. 'It's all about teamwork,' he murmured to me, gesturing around the room at his colleagues.

Now Kostolny got to work. The room was very quiet, the surgeons concentrating intensely, with barely a sound apart from the beeps and whirs of machines. If anyone spoke too loudly, the perfusionist whispered, Martin would not say anything, but might give them a look. Gently, Martin cut away another layer of tissue and started to identify the various parts of the heart. In textbooks they are colour-coded blue and red, but in real life, the heart looks (at least to me) as impenetrable and indistinct as a joint of beef. 'I wouldn't tell the surgeons this,' muttered the perfusionist, 'but they're very clever at what they do.'

At 11, it was time to bypass the heart, so Kostolny could cut into it. The perfusionist's magic machine with no fewer than thirteen separate screens is what makes open heart surgery the success it is today. Not all the screens are critical all the time, but the perfusionist needs to know what's on all of them. The heart-lung machine diverts de-oxygenated blood away from the heart, sends it on a circuit through the machine, where it is oxygenated by an artificial lung, and pumps it back into the heart.

The task most like running a heart-lung machine is flying a plane manually, the smiley chief perfusionist Alex Robertson told me afterwards in his office next to the cardiac theatres, in between cheerful munches of jam on toast prepared in the staff kitchen down the corridor from the operating theatre. 'Like flying a plane, if you stop concentrating, it becomes exciting very quickly,' he laughed. 'We work extremely hard to make it very, very boring.' Alex has worked at GOSH for more than twenty years, and wondered whether he had been at Joel's heart surgery; he even dug the notes out to check. 'No,' he deadpanned, 'the name of the person who stopped your child's heart was Kyrie.'

Alex had left work the previous night at 10 p.m.; he was in again that morning at 6.30. 'The morality of what you're doing is unquestionable,' he told me. 'That makes it easier to drag your sorry carcass into work.' He still hadn't worked out, he added, why he recalls some children and not others. As a perfusionist, he has no real contact with families; the before and the after. 'The operation is the bit they're completely unaware of,' he said. 'We exist in a netherworld of unconsciousness and silence. It's surreal . . . What are we going to do today? We're going to flatline someone.'

Decades ago, the first heart surgeons' challenge was the fact that they could not stop a heart for more than three minutes without causing irreversible brain damage.[18] How could they extend this time, so they could work on the heart for longer? One idea was to bypass the heart. The first primitive attempts in the early 1950s, including a pump circulating a patient's blood through the lungs of four recently killed monkeys in an attempt to oxygenate it, were a tragedy – all five children with tetralogy of Fallot who were subjected to this experiment died.[19]

The other idea was to cool the patient right down. If someone gets lost in the snow for a few hours or is lying apparently dead on a freezing street all night, they are often fine once they are warmed up. (There's a saying in A&E: 'you're not dead until you're warm and dead.') At the start of the twentieth century, operating tables for children were warmed and rooms well heated,[20] but by the middle of the century surgeons were harnessing the fact that the colder you get, the slower your metabolism and the less oxygen and nutrition you need. Cooled down, you can cope better with the reduced blood supply which occurs during an operation, even no blood supply at all for a period. So in the 1950s, anaesthetized patients might be put in a bath filled with crushed ice to cool down, then put on the operating table, where the surgeon would clamp the blood vessels going into the heart, open it up and close the hole in the heart. The heart wouldn't stop – just slow down.

The first successful open heart surgery with a heart-lung machine took place to fix an eighteen-year-old woman's ASD in 1953, and today we have extended the period you can keep the heart stopped to roughly four hours, though even the most complicated cases can expect to spend less than three hours on bypass.[21]

The operating theatre for heart surgery is made as cold as people can bear, wearing disposable paper cardigans. Now, attached to catheters in the child's heart, I watched the heart-lung machine come to life, wide blue plastic tunnels vibrating, tubs of fluid dripping. The heart was still flapping away, beating at its normal rate. It was time to stop it.

Kostolny clamped the aorta, cutting off the blood supply to the coronary artery, effectively the same as inducing a massive heart attack. The moment this was done, they pumped the heart with pleg (pronounced 'pleej'), short for cardioplegia, literally meaning 'still heart' – a solution rich in potassium, which stops the heart. Within about two seconds, I watched the girl's heart rate flatline as it collapsed, empty like a punctured football.

The child was now what people generally consider dead. She had no pulse; her heart was no longer pumping any blood; it had stopped beating. And yet she was very much alive, thanks to the bypass machine. The heart is a shockingly tough organ – it tries to keep going even while a surgeon manhandles it and cuts it.

Only now – a machine doing the work of the heart and lungs, and the heart still and cold so it would not die – could the core operation begin. Heart surgery is essentially a matter of plumbing – rerouting tunnels leading the wrong places, plugging leaks and clearing blocked drains. Mr Kostolny now partially severed the child's aorta and looked down the left ventricle. Now he could remove the tissue that had built up due to the heart's abnormal structure and was blocking the flow from the left ventricle, then suture the aorta back together. He had to do all this without damaging the surrounding valves, the muscles, or the pumping chambers themselves.

Finally, with the heart coping well, the bypass was gradually turned off, after just forty-six minutes. For cardiac surgeons, the best part of the operation is when the heart comes back to life. The longer the heart is clamped and deprived of oxygen, the sicker the patient will be afterwards. This had been relatively short. It was noon, and after phoning to speak with the parents, Kostolny left, telling me he was happy, and that this hadn't been a very complex operation.

At the time I observed, Mr Kostolny was forty-eight. 'Like every other middle-aged man, I have a road bike,' he told me later on, wryly. He likes to cycle in the countryside; he also skis and likes to read 'everything possible'. He grew up in Slovakia, the son of a doctor. Back when he was a final-year medical student, paediatric cardiac surgery was just taking off in Bratislava.

'Were you fascinated by the heart?' I asked.

'That would be too far-fetched,' Martin replied in his quiet, precise voice. 'I guess it's the ability in some cases, by doing complex surgery, to bring a change that immediately leads to a cure. That's not something you can find in many other surgical disciplines. Not in such a dramatic way.'

The day I watched in theatre, after the main operation, there was plenty more for the team to do. For the next two hours, the other surgeons placed the pacemaker and made sure it was set to the right rhythm. Finally, they sewed the chest back up, the scrub nurses having counted every last swab used to make sure nothing had been left inside the body. The physical stamina of everyone involved in the operation was formidable, especially the surgeons and scrub nurses. I was not sure how they managed to stand and focus intently for so many hours, without turning to get a drink, or visit the toilet.

At 1.30 p.m., the drapes were removed. The body, nearly naked again, was illuminated by the bright theatre lights, looking just as it had at the start – no trace of the ordeal it had endured remained other than a neat strip of dressing down the chest and the various drains and tubes. The child, toilet trained already, had come without a nappy; a nurse put one on. They lifted her onto a trolley, covered her with her gown and blankets. Maureen gave her chest a final wipe down. I pulled down my face mask and took a deep breath.

Ellen hand-pumped the ventilator balloon as the girl was wheeled out to the lifts to cardiac intensive care. 'Drive safe,' called the perfusionist.

Up on Flamingo Ward, the child was wheeled into a cubicle; her parents were phoned. As Ellen was briefing the intensive care doctors and nurses, the girl's eyes fluttered and she shifted uncomfortably. It was the moment I myself had dreaded all those times, when consciousness starts to return and the child has to grasp what has happened. The body turned back into a child at this moment. Very quickly, the child's eyes opened fully. She was in obvious distress, trembling, with fear or pain or confusion or all three, I didn't know. My breathing froze. A shot of morphine sent her back under, mercifully. But moments later, she resurfaced, her lips moving, unable to speak while the ventilator covered her nose and filled her lungs. Outside the snow was dizzying. A young Italian nurse with red hair, Chiara, stroked her brow. Later Chiara told me that she would never want to be anything other than an intensive care nurse. 'Shh,' said a doctor, 'good girl . . .' The nurse said: 'You can sleep, sweetie . . . it's all right. Mummy's coming.' The little girl was half awake now, very upset, looking for her parents, trying to cry out, her eyes anxiously darting to everyone's face in vain, but the nurses had to stabilize her first. Another morphine bolus. Now my heart pounded.

The ventilator was clearly uncomfortable and unneeded, so they pulled it out and replaced it with CPAP. The parents – a young couple – arrived, having been told they could come in a little too early. After gazing in initial shock at seeing their daughter like this, the mother moved to her daughter's side and asked if she needed water. The nurses apologetically said it might be best if they left for a few more minutes while they did everything they needed to do. The parents agreed. As the mother let the girl's hand go I saw utter anguish on the child's face. She stretched out her arms to her mother, looked for her desperately. But her mother had to go. Her own face was red and she was sobbing. I held back my own tears.

The stoical girl, who had been here several times before, calmed again. Asked if she was in pain, she shook her head no. Asked if she was OK, she nodded. A nurse put on happy music to distract her: *The Lion Sleeps Tonight*. Then pain gripped her again. She was shaking from head to toe. More morphine. 'We are here to help you, you are not going to be alone,' the nurses told her. They inserted a nasal-gastric tube; she writhed, but it was done fast. Finally her parents could sit with her and hold her hand. I left the room.

It was mid-afternoon. After I changed out of my scrubs (and put the disposable paper cardigan and face mask in my bag for Joel to play doctors with), I walked towards Great Ormond Street's front doors with relief. Upstairs, the staff had hours and hours left of their physically and mentally draining work. And the little girl lay recovering. At the hospital entrance, the mother, on her phone, in tears, walked right past me. I tried to catch her eye, but she didn't recognize me without my scrubs. Out here, in the world.

*

A couple of months after I observed at GOSH, I caught up with Martin Kostolny on the phone to ask a few more questions. What was the patient's prognosis after the operation I observed, I asked? What would her future hold medically?

'Just remind me . . .' he said. 'I don't really have a recollection.'

I looked back over my notes and, relishing trying to sound like a junior doctor, I recounted the facts of the case: 'It was a redo. She'd had an atrioventricular septal defect before that you'd repaired and it had come back with severe subaortic stenosis which was repaired. The operation was to remove an obstruction in her left ventricle. She had also been in heart block and a pacemaker was implanted. Her spleen and stomach were in a slightly odd position . . .' Into the silence as Martin tried to jog his memory, I blurted: 'It was a three-year-old girl . . . blonde plaits . . . it was snowing outside.'

After a pause, Martin chuckled softly. 'I think I vaguely remember.' He does 200 operations a year, and, he explained, 'Usually those who had an uncomplicated post-operative course are more difficult to remember.' When I told him the date, he looked it up on his computer. Now it came back to him.

The child was doing well, but would need to be closely followed up for the rest of her life.

*

To me, Kate Cross will always be 'Miss Cross'.

As for my child, I thought we had explained operations to him as best we could when he was a pre-schooler, but when Joel was seven, he asked me one day as we were getting ready for school: 'What's an operation?'

'It's when a doctor called a surgeon opens up your body to fix a problem inside,' I said.

'How do they open you?' Joel asked.

'Well,' I said, 'first they make you go to sleep – unconscious – so you don't feel anything. And then . . . well, they cut.'

'What with?'

'Um . . . Knives . . . And then they sew you back together again.'

'With what?' Joel asked, disbelievingly.

'Special thread.'

He still looked as if I was telling him a fairy tale, so I told Joel to look down at his own chest. There it was, three years after his heart surgery – a white scar a few inches long. 'They cut open your chest and fixed your heart,' I told him.

He seemed bemused, and that's when it hit me.

I asked Joel: 'Did you not know until now what an operation actually *was*?'

'No'.

Joel knew the word 'operation'; he knew his heart had been fixed; but he had not known – until now – that his body had been cut open with a sharp knife and then sewn back together. Without ever consciously thinking about it, we had shied away from telling him, as a smaller child, that he would be cut open during that euphemistic 'special sleep', let alone that his heart would be stopped. 'Cut' seemed too brutal a word, until both infancy and the operations were long over.

9

Later

'I don't want to be a superhero.'

JOEL

Ever since he was born, my goal had been for Joel to go to the least serious nursery: 'special care'. Finally, in Spring, after recovering from Nissen's fundoplication and gastrostomy surgery, Joel got there.

Phil and I were hospital habitués. We'd got used to living most of our waking hours (in Joel's case, all his life so far) in small corners of wards. But now Joel had had the Nissen's, he could tolerate much more milk – now fed directly into the gastrostomy in his stomach wall – and he stabilized. At last, the rollercoaster started to slow. A day came where we could take Joel out of the neonatal unit for an hour's walk, his first breath of fresh air. I was as anxious as any new mother taking her baby outside for the first time – smearing factor 50 sun cream on him and worrying it wasn't factor 80; adjusting the never-used pram. My mother, Phil and I strolled him to Fitzroy Garden Square, nearby. I wondered if Joel's pale face would light up at seeing outdoors, but he had a quick dreamy look, and fell asleep; it wasn't yet real for him. Then, because Joel was nearly well enough to leave for our local hospital, I was allowed to spend a few days sleeping in a room at UCH, only a floor up from the neonatal unit. Finally I felt something of what it is to be a normal mother. I could see Joel any time of the day or night.

A few weeks later, four months old, Joel went to our local hospital, the Whittington, where that first worrying scan had taken place, for one last month in special care. Here, he was in a large ward where fresh air blew in through open windows, and we could walk him outside for half an hour at a time on a little walkway accessed through the ward. A nurturing neo-natologist, Sharon D'Souza, a new mother herself, doted on him. And then, when it was at long last time to take Joel home, I was allowed to 'room in' with him, sleeping in a little room on the ward with him next to me in a cot. Apart from at Great Ormond Street, I had never spent all night with Joel before and was amazed that he slept solidly, while I prepared and gave him his continuous gastrostomy feeds and medica-tions. At last I let myself dress him in the red sleepsuit with the heart on the tummy, which I'd impulsively bought after my twenty-week scan, during the few weeks I had felt confident in my pregnancy.

He was becoming a little person; every day his gaze seemed more quizzical and whimsical as he took us and the ward in from the white barred cot where he lay flat. There was some-thing playful and yet wistful I saw in my child – he was as sweet yet serious as an old-fashioned gumdrop, I thought. I sang him the strange nursery rhymes that came back to me from my own childhood, like 'Pop Goes the Weasel'. And at last I allowed myself to stop expressing completely, having finally under-stood I could make my life easier and still be a good mother.

On 20 June 2011, five months after his birth, Phil and I were allowed to take Joel home. He had been born in the depths of winter; now it was midsummer. I became a different person in that moment we left hospital behind forever. A happy person, instead of a sad person. And of course Joel changed even more. It was as if in hospital he hadn't been himself; he'd only lived half a life. Suddenly now he came into himself, into his life. A baby, in clothes, out and about, or lying in a Moses basket, rather than a sickly mite in an institutional cot. He fitted into his new life instantly – it was as if he had known nothing else but this homely comfort.

Practically the first thing Phil and I did when we got Joel home was put him in a sling – a sling! Like any other baby – and walk to Cherry Tree Wood.

This was the park we'd talked endlessly to Joel about from his first few days – telling him about the birds and the swings and the squirrels and the sky he would see when he came home. In the photo Phil took of me holding Joel just inside the park, that day, when he finally got to see the sky, the birds and the grass, my mouth is smiling a brand-new happiness but my eyes look haunted. So much had led to that perfect moment, and although it had at last come, it's clear from my eyes I would never forget the path.

*

At last I could get to know my child. A few weeks after coming home, one day lying on the sofa, I saw a mischevious grin and a twinkle in Joel's eye as he kicked his legs proud and high. It was as if I recognized him for the first time. Here he was – this was Joel, I instantly knew.

Coming out of hospital was like being set free from prison. I couldn't bear to look at the blankets and finger puppets and musical mobile Joel had had in hospital – I gave away almost everything we'd bought for him in the early months. I went

shopping with Grace, now Joel's godmother (her gamely holding a crying Joel while I ran around throwing garments into
his buggy to try on); I went to baby yoga; I met friends and
their babies in cafes – me tube-feeding Joel while they fed their
babies purée. But life was never really 'normal'.

Joel had two paediatricians (general and developmental), a
cardiologist, physiotherapist, dietician and a speech and language therapist (the last two to get him to eat, in the face of
severe reflux and an oral aversion – although the Nissen's
stopped him vomiting and aspirating, the underlying retching
and discomfort of reflux remained, and babies who are tube-
fed for a long time lose the instinct to eat and drink using their
mouths). He also had a rather severe Eastern European gastrostomy nurse, and a sweetly bustling young district nurse
who visited at least weekly. We called the group 'Team J'.

Phil and I acquired nursing skills. Every Sunday after Joel's
bath, we had to do what felt like a mini-operation. We'd lie
Joel on our bed on a clean towel and I'd distract him with toys.
Meanwhile Phil would insert an empty syringe into Joel's gastrostomy button and drain out the balloon of water under his
skin which, when inflated, kept the button in place. Very
swiftly, Phil then had to fill the balloon again with fresh water,
while holding the button securely with his other hand. If the
button popped out of Joel, he would have an open hole in his
stomach, and its contents could pour out. If left without the
button for a few minutes, we were told, the hole might seal
shut and Joel would need another operation to cut it open
again. So we rushed through this procedure at home against
the clock.

Every morning Phil measured Joel's array of medications
into the correct doses in syringes, about ten of them each day,
ready to inject into his gastrostomy at set intervals. There was

medicine to help his reflux; to repair his bones fractured by metabolic bone disease; to stop his heart going into meltdown; viscous red iron to avoid anaemia. His prescription formula, feeding pump and syringes were delivered, all paid for by the NHS, every few weeks in huge boxes.

In the daytimes, we dribbled 'bolus' feeds of formula very slowly into a plungerless syringe attached to Joel's gastrostomy, and at night he was hooked up to a feeding pump which dripped the milk into his stomach continuously for twelve hours, from 9 p.m. to 9 a.m. This gradual feeding was the only way to get enough calories into him – he was too refluxy to manage much at a time.

One night Phil had to go away for work, so my parents came to fill in for him. Their main task was taking over what Phil usually did at 4 a.m., which was making up a fresh formula feed to run on Joel's feeding pump for the next five hours, and setting it up on the pump. Phil – an early bird naturally waking up at 4 a.m. anyway – was a pro at this routine, and his doing it meant I got to stay asleep at this time, before Joel woke me around 6 a.m. I thought my mother would find it just as easy, since she, like Phil, is a very early riser.

In the evening, I gave her a tutorial in pump feeding, showing her how it all worked – by that time, it seemed very simple to me, just a matter of unscrewing a plastic container, turning a dial and pressing a few clearly labelled buttons.

At 4 a.m., my bedroom door creaked loudly open. 'It's us!' Mum whispered very loudly. She'd brought Dad along to help her. They stumbled into the room and continued their discussion in increasingly urgent whispers. 'OK, so I unscrew this bit, and put in this – oh no, that's not right . . . no, no, it's this dial. No! Not that way – THAT way! Right, so I turn this to three o'clock. And then this to eleven o'clock. No, that's not working. Where does this bit go? I can't see a thing.'

I lay there, listening to Joel's breathing change as all the activity started to wake him up. Then, forgetting we had a lovely, effective little nightlight, Mum turned on the overhead light. I buried my head into the pillow.

The light went off again, then suddenly on again. 'Where's the bathroom light?' Mum and Dad wondered aloud as they flicked different overhead lights on and off until the bedroom looked like a disco.

'I'll take over now!' I muttered, getting up to sort out the lights and supervise the turning of the dial and pressing of buttons. Half a minute later, all was set up and the pump was running nicely, Joel was sleeping, and I was ushering my poor bumbling parents out of the bedroom, feeling bad for getting cross when they were only trying to help. And of course it was dark, and their eyesight was not as good as mine, and they weren't used to setting the pump. And they must have been very tired, too.

I felt so guilty that I couldn't get back to sleep, and tossed and turned for an hour. The next night, I sent them home to get a good night's sleep and did the 4 a.m. pump job by myself. What a relief, all round.

Of course, my parents were in fact not bumblers, but on the contrary, extraordinarily helpful and capable. Dad noticed things we needed in the house, like the endless supply of paper plates required to put Joel's syringes on, and he stocked up for us at the supermarket without us having to think about it. As a doctor, he also continued to explain medical issues to us, always reassuringly. My mother was the only person besides Phil and me who learned how to give Joel his tube feeds and vent his gastrostomy to burp him. She helped me bathe Joel, then straightened my bed and folded some laundry.

A natural storyteller, she had her own animated style of telling Joel a favourite Winnie-the-Pooh story – the one where Pooh gets stuck in Rabbit's burrow – with a joyful emphasis on how 'all Rabbit's friends and relations' tugged and tugged until, 'POP!' – Pooh was free. She talked and sang and connected with Joel all the time. And as a mother herself, she thought of things no one else did, not even the professionals. For instance, that it would work for me to try to breastfeed Joel at the same time as giving him a tube feed – that way he was calmer and associated feeding with his stomach getting full, and we weren't struggling to fit in one before the other.

After we took Joel home, I found that the extremity of my initiation into motherhood had pushed me to a point where I wasn't going to take any more crap.

As a new mother, I remembered what it felt like to be a child – the indignation at being told what to do all the time, feeling patronized, insignificant and powerless. From being accused of wetting myself when my waters broke to the refusal of an extra blanket the night after giving birth to being called 'mum' (just as I had once hated being called 'kid') to the prying bossiness of health visitors, motherhood was the first time since I was a schoolgirl that I had felt so small.

I saw how mothers can be guilt-tripped into performing certain laborious and tedious tasks and buying certain products. Tsk! Tsk! emanates from expensive packaging. '70 per cent of mothers have an undersheet alarm – protect against the risk of cot death.' So much of motherhood is about the risk of death – the need to buy brand-new mattresses and car seats is gospel. By the time Joel came home, I had spent so much time living with a high chance of death that I was determined, now he was essentially well, to keep danger in proportion. So I didn't buy the undersheet which alarmed if the baby stopped breathing. Joel had slept over one in hospital at Great Ormond Street, and I knew how often a false alarm was triggered when he was actually breathing. It was time to stop scaring myself unnecessarily. The NICU had given me an acute sense of proportion. Now, every time I heard a mother fretting about her baby's trauma at being immunized, I couldn't help but think: 'You have no idea.'

There is something of the martyr in motherhood, I found, that makes women feel guilty if they admit they would really rather not spend precious hours of the day (and night) doing dull menial tasks such as cleaning breast pumps, then carefully airdrying them to ensure they are ready for the next expressing session. And there is something of the finger-wagging matron in the companies which peddle these products to mothers, with their many fussy little rules on the correct use of nipple correctors, how to fill a sterilizer with exactly X millilitres of water (no more, no less), and that products cannot be put in the dishwasher. A dishwasher would make it all too easy and convenient. The mother must scrub things with a special brush. Well, I replied to Medela and Nuk's packaging in my head after Joel came home, neonatologist Dr Giles Kendall told me to wash your products in the dishwasher and they are just fine!

Thankfully the melodic words of our favourite Welsh valleys neonatal nurse now rang in my ears: 'Ev-er-y ba-by is an indi-VID-u-AL.' That stood me in good stead when, at last beginning some semblance of ordinary parenting, I discovered the baby books which dictated a rigid timetable not only for the baby, but for the mother herself: when the mother should eat breakfast, the exact half-hour when she is allowed some time for herself. Baby must be changed and ready for the day by 7 a.m. and no later!

There was one piece of so-called 'advice' I'd been given – and seen given to other mothers – from early in my pregnancy onwards. The usually unsolicited advice goes along the lines of: 'Stop worrying, otherwise it's going to affect your baby.' It was, I came to realize, perhaps the single most patronizing, counter-productive thing modern mothers get told.

The advice was given to me many times by well-meaning neonatal nurses, including one who, on finding me crying quietly by the incubator one day, told me to leave the room, presumably so I didn't upset Joel, or perhaps so I didn't upset anyone else. A registrar at Great Ormond Street gave the advice to me too. I was having a discussion with her about administrative problems in this particular department concerning Joel's records – the kind of thing any parent is likely to get frustrated about. The registrar meant well and promised to sort the problems out, but she ended the discussion by saying to me sternly: 'Look, you must not let yourself get stressed about this, otherwise Joel will sense it and it will upset him.' My cowed response? 'Of course, doctor.'

If you are a stressed mother-to-be or mother, the worst thing you can be told is that your stress is going to adversely affect your baby; maybe even cause a miscarriage. Far from helping a mother to relax, this 'advice' only makes her more worried and insecure. I couldn't just 'stop' feeling stressed – it was not a button I could switch off. I had learned now that if Joel did sense me being genuinely stressed, I sensed his love and concern for me. The fact that he picked up on my emotions wasn't a problem or my fault in some way; we simply loved each other. My maternal instinct had been vulnerable to being undermined by authority, but by the end of my time in the NICU, I had regained trust in myself.

I decided I was going to be a mother who refused to live her life by a school-like timetable because she was capable of making her own decisions and loved freedom and knew deep within her what was right for her baby. Becoming a mother in the neonatal unit was a trial by fire, but I'd learned a lot.

*

'You haven't fixed it just because they've gone home,' Joel's neonatal consultant Judith Meek once told me. Hospital is only the first step for these survivors. And there's no precedence, no road map for this new generation.

When Joel couldn't breathe unaided in hospital, I'd wondered how other babies knew how to breathe, and now, I wondered how others just got up and walked. At his first Christmas party, nearly a year old, he lay beached on the floor in a Santa onesie – unable to sit up unsupported, while the other babies his age already crawled and toddled. Joel had hours of physiotherapy to do 'tummy time' even for a moment. He first crawled when he was about fifteen months corrected,[†] and was so excited that night I saw him crawling in his sleep.

Joel was tiny, physically fragile and tired easily. He didn't want to make marks on paper; he clutched crayons so awkwardly it was impossible. I got used to strangers assuming Joel was half his age. When he was nine months old, people

---

† A premature-born infant's 'corrected' age is their chronological age minus the number of months they were born early. So Joel, born two months early, was fifteen months 'corrected' when he was seventeen months old. Correcting age is a fairer way to measure a premature baby's milestones.

had complimented me on my newborn. Later, a well-meaning man who saw Joel whizzing around with his baby walker asked me, 'Is he one yet?'

'Actually, he's two,' I replied.

Joel was two-and a half when he took his first steps unaided. Even then, his movements were tense and angular; I often felt his little heart beating fast with anxiety and frustration. Nothing came easily.

Understandably, given his gastrostomy tube poking out of his sensitive reflux stomach, Joel did not like being roly-polyed down my legs at baby yoga. And he cried in cafes and at music groups. In fact, he cried much of the time for his first two years.

No one in 'Team J' could tell us why. We were assured it couldn't be connected to the gastrostomy, and anyway, that couldn't come out until he learned to eat and drink, or he would starve. So at playgroups and friends' houses, I would watch other children play while I held a sobbing child, often in tears myself. I didn't find out what was wrong until just before Joel's second birthday.

Joel had finally mastered eating and drinking orally. A specialist nurse whisked out his gastrostomy button in seconds, just like that. Joel changed too, just like that. The near-constant crying stopped. And then I realized that my son, who didn't yet have words to tell us what was bothering him so much, had found the gastrostomy extremely uncomfortable. And, after the nonstop interventions during his five months in hospital, he had had to endure this constant irritation for more than eighteen months of his life.

The stomach problems continued until Joel was three, because the open wound left by the gastrostomy button didn't close naturally, as expected. Whenever Joel caught a cold, his digestive system ground to a halt and stomach acid jetted out from the bandage over the wound, stinging painfully across his skin; in effect a chemical burn. Flummoxed A&E staff (we regularly seemed to end up hanging out with them on Saturday nights) experimented with all kinds of alternative bandages to try to cover the wound, often leaving Joel's torso wrapped up like a mummy, but the stomach acid seeped through any dressing.

The wound around the gastrostomy never healed. Instead, sore red tissue circled the hole, and a constant procession of district nurses came to our house to try to kill this granulation tissue with wands tipped with silver nitrate that made Joel scream as they burned his skin. In the end, Joel had to have two more operations under general anaesthetic to seal the hole and heal the tissue around it.

So, make that three years of discomfort Joel endured. By the time of his open heart surgery at age four, he had had an operation every year of his life, and one before birth, of course. So it was hardly surprising that Joel was an over-sensitive pre-schooler. When the wind blew, he quaked. When he heard a loud noise – a hand dryer or a balloon popping, for instance – he flat-out panicked. Certain simple sensations which might at most annoy another child – brushing hair, face washing, pulling a jumper over his head, setting foot on sand – were not routine for Joel.

It wasn't that he was unhappy. He was always ready to cuddle, yabbered excitedly nonstop using made-up words like 'rowley cake' which Phil and I could never interpret, and nothing could distract him from his beloved toy vehicles. But there were many tiny little things which he resisted: when I pushed his buggy in the woods he cried, upset by the bumpy ground. A shower after swimming was another cause of terror.

Even a colourful scarf or parachute handed to him at a play-group to hold wasn't straightforward: he wouldn't hold on to it and would wriggle in my lap and cry. New things seemed frightening for him. While some sensations bothered him, he craved others – he chewed his clothes and loved to cuddle and stroke other people and clothes, especially fluffy materials.

When he was two or three, children his age, some almost twice his height and weight, would brush past him and knock him to the floor without even noticing. A little fall left him shocked and crying, while most others his age wouldn't topple in the first place, and if they did, they would jump up again without a whimper. At the adventure playground one day a boy exactly Joel's age climbed up an enormous twisty slide and hurtled down it. Joel could only stand holding my hand, watching, amazed – he could not so much as climb the steps alone.

At nursery, the other children were protective of Joel, treating him like a cross between a younger child and a celebrity. When he arrived each afternoon his friends would line up to greet him, pet him and feed him, and watch him whizz off with his baby walker. Characteristically – and perhaps why they adored him – Joel didn't even notice their adulation: he just wanted to play. 'Box of cars?' he would say expectantly, every time he entered a room. The staff had to explain to his peers that he was actually the same age as them. I was touched but I also worried about what school might be like for Joel when other children weren't so sweet. Especially because he was a boy, and it's not easy in this world to be a small, fragile male.

Although the extreme crying of Joel's first two years ended with the removal of the gastrostomy, he still cried more than the average toddler. He also struggled to sit still and listen. Waiting in a queue, mild hunger, not having my full attention – any small stress could send him into meltdown – and eventually I realized that emotional self-regulation, the root feeling of OK-ness most of us take for granted, was something he would have to acquire, because it was not built in for Joel as it is for most people. Along with the coordination needed to hold a pencil, to jump in the air, not to trip over his own feet.

Before starting school Joel had to give answers to a list of questions about himself. One was 'What are you good at?' His response, which I dutifully wrote down for him, was: 'Having operations'. In his first year of school, Joel seemed lost. In class, he found it hard to sit and be quiet at circle time. He clutched his pencil in his fist and wept with frustration at not being able to mark down on paper what was in his head. And he chewed his clothes and those of other children, and stroked children's hair. Everyone understood, thanks to the magic words 'special needs' – except one girl's parents, who looked at him with disgust, while I apologized for Joel's love of their daughter's silky hair. The mother didn't notice Joel reaching out to stroke her fake fur gilet even as she gazed with her lip curled at him, and I didn't think it wise to draw her attention to it. There were so many labels, so many names, I learned, for overlapping differences in a young child's behaviour: autism, ADHD, sensory processing disorder, auditory processing disorder, dyspraxia, developmental delay. Whatever you wanted to call it, Joel was wired just a little differently. He was not 'neurotypical'.

Being different is a gift society is only just learning to value. Joel's originality and sensitivity were also his strengths. From his earliest days, we had observed his soulfulness and seriousness, and as he grew up he displayed a philosophical curiosity about life and a deeply loving and affectionate nature. He had no toughness, no hard edge or malice. When I was sad, he noticed immediately and rushed to hug and comfort me. He would start conversations with anybody – asking a grumpy builder in a caff, 'And then you will have pudding?' and a young woman on a bus, 'Hello, what is your name called? What is your favourite reptile?'

He also had no dullness. Bright and eager, he yearned at four and five and six to understand ideas like infinity, reality and death, as well as maintaining passionate interests in, for instance, jellyfish and fungi. He never cared too much what others thought of him – he was joyfully himself. When people met Joel, they remembered him. He had spirit; joie de vivre. There was something almost magically, heartbreakingly inno-cent about his keenness to play and have toys; forever young like Peter Pan. As he got older and could express more, he begged me never to say the word 'death'. His sole wish, when a teacher asked him, was 'to live forever'. He became horrified after seeing an illustration in a book of an aged human, stooped over, leaning on a stick. 'Will I lean?' Joel asked Phil and me again and again.

Painstakingly he learned what he needed to, and most importantly, how to feel 'OK' – he did everything late, but, as with the breathing in hospital and learning to eat and drink, he got there. Again and again we were stunned by how sud-denly he developed. When he was five, I worried he would never be able to draw a circle. One Saturday at the age of six and a half he got up and wrote and illustrated an eighty-page book about poisonous mushrooms, the names, like 'fly agaric', huge and wobbly across a whole page. He discovered he loved to junk model, imagine he was flying to Mars ('and home in time for tea'), and hunt for deadly adders in the garden.

By the age of six and a half, Joel had stopped chewing other children's clothes (if not his own), was fine with taking showers and had even learned not to panic at the hand dryer at school, although elsewhere, dryers made public toilets a nightmare for him. Still, he struggled to learn to sit down if he was tired and not to call out the first thing that came to his mind. Impractical and unaware of his environment, he needed help with basic tasks like turning handles and couldn't catch a ball. Medical check-ups and vaccinations remained frightening for him. At his appointments he was afraid when the blood pressure cuff inflated around his arm, or when he had a heart scan, no matter how much I explained that the operations were all over and that no one was going to hurt him. 'What are they doing to my heart?' he cried at one heart echo. 'Am I going to have an operation?' he would ask before every routine check-up. He nestled into my arms as fragile and wild as a bird.

Undoubtedly, many of Joel's early challenges can be linked to having Noonan syndrome, but Phil and I – as well as his doctors – always had a gut feeling that his intense medical start in life also greatly affected his development. How could it not?

I first realized we were not alone when I came across an article online about a two-year-old American boy called Elijah. In 'science fiction' open fetal surgery at CHOP, Scott Adzick had removed a tumour the size of an orange from Elijah's left lung. He was then born seven weeks premature. Elijah's mother April's description of her son as a little boy sounded just like Joel. 'Giving him a bath was so difficult, and changing his diaper was so hard. He would cry and scream. Everything new was hard for him to adapt to . . . Meeting new people. Trying new things. The wind in his face. The snow in his hands.' April added, 'I don't know if it's because of everything he's been through or if it's just who he is.'[1] It could have been me talking.

Not long after Joel came home, I read the journalist David Aaronovitch's account of recovery in intensive care in a London hospital from keyhole surgery to remove a pre-cancerous growth in his colon.[2] 'I will never forget those days and nights of terror and delusion,' he wrote. Aware of tubes all over his body, breathing with a mask at times, tube-fed, he struggled with the desire to cough up the tube in his throat and was tormented by thirst and nausea. For several days, he suffered from delusions in which the nurses were attacking and trying to kill him. After he recovered, he learned that ICU psychosis, a horrible blend of hallucinations and paranoia, can affect as many as one third of intensive care patients. It is an understandable response to being physically helpless: drugged, tubed, in pain. If a grown man can go through this horror during a few days in intensive care, what is the potential impact for a baby whose first months are lived solely in intensive care or high dependency?

If you believe that a person's sense of being – the way they feel for the rest of their life – is to some degree formed and shaped by their earliest experiences – ideally being held safely by their mother – then the reverse must also be true: a baby who is separated physically from its mother at birth and raised for months in a plastic box, tortured in effect by endless medical procedures, can be expected to become overwhelmed by sensations and emotions, to struggle to feel secure. A growing body of research suggests that the harsh neonatal unit experience can affect some children's neurological development, potentially causing difficulties with sensory processing, behaviour and learning as they grow up.

The guinea-pig millennial generation of NICU survivors

have spent their first months in what one neonatalogist described to me as 'a horrible environment where they had a lot of invasive things done'. The new generation of young people whose lives have been made possible by modern medicine are growing up with previously untreatable problems like hypoplastic left heart syndrome; since the 1980s and 1990s we have the first survivors of extreme prematurity, whose lives are now the subject of increasing study. These young survivors have often undergone significant levels of trauma in their first months. Modern medicine is still getting to grips with the long-term developmental impact of spending one's earliest months – before and after birth – undergoing intensive medical interventions.

In the uterus there isn't a lot of sensory stimulus, and we now know that over-stimulating immature babies in the brightly lit, noisy, busy NICU might change their neurological development: for example, small premature babies respond to touch in the same way as pain. Touch – perceived as pain – affects their central nervous system and in turn their neurological development.[3] One review of a number of studies reported that in NICU babies born at thirty-two weeks or earlier, the life-saving stream of painful medical interventions to which they were subjected was associated with altered brain development, the programming of the body's stress systems and pain perceptions later in life. Conditioned to repeated and unpredictable pain/stress, without the constant cuddling and soothing a baby at home receives, a NICU baby who has a heel prick test shows signs of stress thirty minutes later when their nappy is changed. To make matters worse, a preterm baby cannot yet physically regulate their heightened responses to pain, and the expectation of continual pain and stress may be programmed into their developing brain's synaptic connections and cortical networks which control its function.[4] I only had to look at my son as he grew older to witness this. Joel was hypersensitive; he was often flooded with stress and did not seem to have an inbuilt ability to self-soothe. For a long time, he continued to become upset very easily, even by insignificant things like the wind blowing or a tiny stumble.

EPICure, a ground-breaking British study, has been tracking the long-term effects of extreme prematurity on children as they grow up, and has reported that around two in three such children need some help at school, with difficulty paying attention common, and just over one in four has behaviour problems. Some of these children display signs of autism, but this is different from classic autism.[5] There may be a unique kind of rewiring involving traits of autism and/or ADHD particular to some children whose early months were spent, perhaps premature, in hospital.

Incubators have been described as 'neurodevelopmental dungeons' by one Harvard University paediatrician.[6] 'We should all bear in mind these babies are actually fetuses,' Dr Amir Lahav has said. 'The intensive care unit is a noisy place with electronic and digital sounds which the baby would not get in a room, or white noise. If the primary stimulation that you are exposed to is white noise . . . you are essentially teaching your brain . . . to perceive noise in the foreground not the background. Let's fast forward to third grade and you have a child struggling to attend to what the teacher is saying because his brain was not wired in a way to concentrate on a human voice.' When I read that, I thought of Joel – how although there was nothing wrong with his ability to hear, he found it hard to listen in any noisy, busy place. The sound of a group of people talking seemed to cause him physical discomfort; it appeared too loud for him – and it masked his ability to attend to what any one person was saying. To him, it was just an onslaught of unpleasant sound that didn't make sense, like trying to listen to multiple foreign radio stations at the same time at top volume.

Of course Joel was not extremely premature, but even without prematurity, time in hospital alone has also been found to have an effect on babies – long stays in intensive care and major surgery early in life have been linked with later difficulties with learning, memory, motor skills, mental health and 'executive function' – the mental processing control that allows us to get tasks done.[7]

Not only hospitals but schools, too, are starting to understand the particular special needs of pupils born premature, or sick. 'Many have learning difficulties that have not previously been encountered,' wrote Professor Barry Carpenter, an SEN expert and former headteacher, in an education journal. 'It is my belief that we as teachers must develop new generation pedagogy for this new generation of children.' In his view, autistic traits in children born very premature are 'an attachment-based autism, perhaps stemming from the fact that you cannot hold, stroke or smile at your baby if they are in an incubator as you could if they are in your arms.'[8] As well as being clumsy and under-confident, prem-born children, he noted, may be 'hyper-vigilant and hyper-aroused' and find planning ahead and organizing difficult.

I believe all this applies equally to a child like Joel who, though not born very premature, spent his first five months in hospital and his first three years in physical discomfort. So when Joel came last in the races at school sports day (heart-warmingly finishing to the sound of all the older children cheering his name), or meandered his lost way around birthday parties covering his ears as others danced and popped balloons, I kept thinking how Joel had already endured far more in his earliest months and years than all those strapping, healthy children around him.

To take just one example, my son had a tube stabbed into his chest in utero without anaesthetic. I was given local anaesthetic for my abdomen. Phil and I asked, beforehand, whether the baby would be anaesthetized too – after all, he was about to have a long needle stuck, presumably pretty painfully, through his chest wall – and what if he moved suddenly and the needle went in the wrong place? But as we understood it, that hazy day, it just wasn't done. We accepted the protocol – there was no other option.

I later asked around and found out that anaesthetic is usually only given to fetuses undergoing longer procedures (like open fetal surgery or a balloon for congenital diaphragmatic hernia). Unbelievably, the idea that even a newborn baby in hospital, let alone a fetus, could feel pain, has only been recognized medically since the 1980s. Before then, doctors assumed young babies could not perceive pain.[9] Now we know they do, yet all the fetal medics I have spoken to have told me that they don't anaesthetize the fetus for procedures like a shunt because it's a quick procedure the baby won't remember. They seemed bemused by me even questioning it. There is an issue with giving analgesics to a fetus, too: the worry that a developing brain might not respond well to drugs – an anaesthetic could be potentially more harmful than the fetus enduring a sharp pain for a moment. It would also mean an additional injection through the mother's uterus, which would increase the risk of miscarriage.

I have the utmost respect for what fetal doctors do. Yet as a mother, I can't help wondering if in future we could find a different way. A doctor wouldn't stick a shunt into a twenty-nine-week-old neonate's chest without pain relief, but surely

it's an equally painful experience for a baby of the same gestation in utero.

*

Gillian Kennedy was Joel's first speech and language therapist
in the NICU. You might wonder why a neonate needs speech
and language therapy, but in the neonatal unit, these clinicians
focus not on language but on the most basic oral skill: encour-
aging babies to suck and swallow milk. Phil and I were struck
by the graceful balletic way this slim woman with cropped
grey hair moved and her super-soft baby-friendly voice; how
gently she approached Joel.

Years later, as I observed on a warm March day in a high
dependency neonatal ward at UCH, Gillian opened an incubator, and murmured softly: 'Hello, little bean. Look at you,
you snuggly person.'

Baby William had been born three weeks before, at twenty-
six weeks' gestation, and was breathing with the help of a
CPAP machine. On the whiteboard next to his incubator, a
nurse had written: 'minimal handling'. For all premature
babies, being in neonatal care is extremely stressful, and nurses
had observed that William seemed especially unsettled when
they did his 'cares'.

Kennedy was there to find out 'what William is telling those
caring for him – and to learn from him what challenges him
as well as noting his own efforts to settle himself'. She watched
his breathing closely and observed patterns of shallow breaths
followed by a faster breath and then a shuddery stretch.

William's tiny movements pointed to him trying to breathe
more easily. It seemed, Kennedy thought, that William needed
extra time to adjust to being touched or slower handling. He

might have been experiencing discomfort connected to his breathing efforts or digestion, or caused by overstimulation – too much noise, light and sudden physical contact.

'Are you all right?' Gillian suddenly asked me. 'Yes, fine,' I said. 'Just some acid indigestion.' I had barely been conscious of it myself, but Gillian had noticed I was showing signs of the slightest refluxy discomfort. It's what she is trained to do.

She is now helping run the British training centre at UCH for NIDCAP, the person-centred philosophy of neonatal care which I observed being practised in Stockholm, which aims to give a voice to these most fragile of babies. NIDCAP tries to make the neonatal unit experience less stressful by following a baby's cues, attending to each infant as an individual. Nurses following the NIDCAP approach 'listen' and adjust their care for babies in the same way that they would for an older child who speaks and makes their likes and dislikes known.

There's nothing fluffy about NIDCAP, by the way – it has concrete effects on medical outcomes. Babies treated under NIDCAP come off ventilators faster, have a reduced chance of chronic lung disease and are discharged from neonatal units earlier. And at follow-up, the child has more organized behaviour, especially in terms of visual-spatial ability and motor planning.[10]

At another high dependency incubator, Gillian noticed a thirty-one-week-old girl's legs flailing. She arranged for an extra muslin blanket to gently contain them – or 'snuggle her in', as she put it – while a staff nurse placed both hands on the baby to soothe her. The baby's blood oxygen saturation rose as she calmed.

I watched nurses trained in the approach gain a baby's 'permission' before a procedure by waiting, wherever possible, until the baby woke naturally, giving them time to settle, and softly, respectfully explaining what was about to happen. They moved the baby slowly and smoothly, adjusting to their responses before holding them under still hands for as long as necessary to give comfort before, during and after a procedure. One nurse or doctor might focus on performing a procedure while another nurse focuses completely on comforting the baby. Blood tests or even lumbar punctures can be done while the baby rests on his mother's chest. Unnatural noise, bright light and sudden touch on the ward are kept to a minimum.

UCH staff sister and neonatal nurse educator Jenny Montague told me the NIDCAP approach can be challenging. 'For some of us it comes instinctively, but for others it doesn't. A lot of nursing jobs are very task-oriented, and nurses like to do things quickly, but babies don't always like that. When a baby is holding his hand out he might be asking, "Where am I?" or saying, "I don't like this, go away." Move slowly and see how he responds to you when you go at his pace.'

The tsunami of new advances which had established neonatal care was ebbing by the late 1990s. The focus has since shifted. UCH neonatal consultant Professor Neil Marlow, director of the new NIDCAP centre and expert on the long-term effects of prematurity, believes neonatal care is evolving into a new era: 'When we started, we were trying to save lives. We've got good at that. What we now need to do is look at the quality of that survival.' Research on this is still in its infancy, but Professor Marlow told me that the outlook for the first extremely premature generation is 'remarkably upbeat'. Professor Marlow told me: 'As time's gone on, we've shown that for a lot of children who had difficult neonatal periods, that's the only problem they have. For others there is more of a problem and it's difficult to predict what's going to happen.'

He noted: 'Many of the kids who had obvious problems at eleven have adjusted well over adolescence and become high-functioning adults. And a lot of the problems with attention seem to have disappeared [by nineteen].'[11] It's also worth noting that a baby treated in a high level neonatal unit — like Joel — is likely to have a better outcome.

It's interesting how many babies who start their lives with months in the NICU develop normally, without any problems. As fetal and neonatal medicine have evolved, 'medical miracles' increasingly not only survive, but live totally normal lives, often with extraordinary achievements.

Ben Wills, from the Wirral, was one of the first babies in Britain to be saved at twenty-three weeks' gestation back in 1990, weighing a healthy 907 grams, after his mother developed a burst abscess on her appendix. He was one of the first premature babies in the UK to receive surfactant. At school, Ben got top marks in exams and excelled at sports. Today, six feet tall and a writer, he has degrees in archaeology and physiology, has written a book about neonatology, and campaigns for Bliss, the premature baby charity. Although for his first six months he was deaf, Ben has had perfect hearing since.

Others born sick have a tougher path, with developmental, learning, sensory, physical or behavioural differences that are still barely understood. I watched my friends' 'miracle' children grow up – either, like Joel, at mainstream schools with one-on-one support, or at special schools – and noticed how similar they were in their differences, despite no two having the same diagnosis.

Confident, strong Eve's extremely premature son Noah, whom she hadn't been able to hold until he was nearly eight weeks old, came home on oxygen and a nasogastric tube. He had spent the same length of time as Joel – the first five months – in hospital, and like Joel had endured a life-and-death rollercoaster including neonatal surgery. As they became toddlers and pre-schoolers, it was impossible not to notice similarities in the way Noah and Joel differed from other children. Although he grew big and strong physically, Noah was, just like Joel, an emotionally fragile young boy. Noah would often 'scream the place down' or vomit, apparently terrified, especially when anyone other than his parents Eve and Charlie approached him. They felt they 'couldn't take him anywhere' – and picked times to take him to the park when nobody else was around, never after school or on weekends. The crying improved, but during his childhood, Noah, in his little blue spectacles – his eyesight affected by retinopathy of prematurity – continued to be sensitive and had ups and downs with various difficulties in sensory processing (for example fearing loud noises), 'as well as concentration, learning, speech, eating and fine and gross motor skills,' Eve reeled off to me, as a special needs parent gets used to doing.

A likely reason for Noah's anxiety was obvious to Eve as an occupational therapist and psychotherapist, as it was to me. Our sons were almost certainly traumatized, lacking a fundamental sense of security. Some symptoms classified under ADHD or autism – for instance high 'reactivity' – might in fact be symptoms of post-traumatic stress in neonatal unit survivors. A much-loved preterm baby's inevitable experience of over-stimulation, pain and parental separation in the NICU can be as traumatic as the experience of a baby who is neglected or abused. (No wonder one mother of a NICU baby told me the unit reminded her, strangely, of a Romanian orphanage.) Eve chose a mainstream school and – a woman who was not afraid to think differently – neither pursued nor accepted diagnoses of autism and ADHD for Noah: she did not want him labelled because she feared this might limit others' (and even his own) view of his potential. She found Noah a specialist psychotherapist and tried to work on what she saw as the cause of his different behaviour – stress and anxiety.

Of course Noah had also undergone another major ordeal at the start of life – he had lost his twin. Again, the potential trauma of such an experience at the beginning of a life has yet to be recognized, though some have believed in it. At the dawn of the 1980s, the Italian psychiatrist Alessandra Piontelli was asked to see an eighteen-month-old boy who was behaving slightly strangely. Jacob was an intelligent infant who was driving his parents mad with incessant restlessness and lack of sleep. Piontelli noticed how he moved as if 'obsessed by a search for something in every possible corner of the limited space of my consulting room, looking for something which he never seemed able to find . . . occasionally Jacob also tried to shake several of the objects inside my room, as if trying to bring them back to life.'

When the doctor observed that Jacob appeared to be looking for something or someone he had lost, his parents burst into tears. They explained that Jacob was in fact a twin, whose brother, Tino, had died two weeks before birth. Jacob had spent two weeks in utero with his dead and unresponsive brother.

Piontelli believed that traumatic experience continued to affect Jacob's infancy. This experience prompted the psychiatrist to the belief that a fetus in the womb has a rudimentary psychological awareness. With the new technology of ultrasound available in the 1980s, she started her research observing babies' behaviour while being scanned in utero, and then after birth, finding that in many cases, 'personalities' seemed to be notable well before birth.[12] As Sigmund Freud wrote, 'There is much more continuity between intra-uterine life and earliest infancy than the impressive caesura of the act of birth would have us believe.'[13]

As for Allie, my unpretentious, clever friend whose twins Beth and Emily were born at twenty-five weeks, the road ahead was to be harder than she imagined in the weeks after birth. After two months progressing well in the high-level neonatal unit in London, and neurosurgery for Beth following her haemorrhage, when Beth's hand was the size of Allie's fingernail, the twins were both off CPAP and on high-flow oxygen, just tiny nasal prongs rather than a mask. They were well enough to be sent to their local hospital, in the north of England – but from that moment on, the situation unravelled.

Re-ventilated and sedated, the girls were airlifted to the other hospital. Having a tube in the airways is an infection risk, and that day both girls picked up infections. Emily had been doing well, but the infection proved a massive blow. She couldn't breathe with just high-flow oxygen any more. She was back on the dreaded CPAP. Emily seemed an unhappy child, Allie thought at the time – she refused to feed and cried all the time. After six months on CPAP, Emily had to have a tracheostomy – a breathing tube inserted through a hole in the windpipe – so she could finally go home. (Without the trachy, which allowed her to use CPAP through a tube in her throat, Emily would have had to remain on facial CPAP, with a mask over her face at all times.) After the tracheostomy, Emily changed immediately into a happy, uncomplaining child. It was then that Allie realized just how uncomfortable the facial CPAP had been for Emily. Later, doctors found a heart defect between Emily's aorta and pulmonary artery called a patent ductus arteriosus (PDA), which could well have caused the breathing trouble. It was repaired, but damage had been done.

In the end, Beth was in neonatal care for four and a half months; Emily, who had promisingly managed to come off the oscillating ventilator after a week to everyone's joy, was in neonatal care for ten months. Emily's lungs sustained long-term damage from the long periods of ventilation and CPAP. When I first met her, and she was six, Emily still desaturated several times a night and needed oxygen at home if she got a cold.

For Allie, as hard as the time in hospital was, the toughest thing by far was the realization, as years passed, that her children would have lifelong disabilities.

The way the girls' disabilities developed was surprising. Emily was the sickly one in the neonatal period, coming home with a tracheostomy, which she had until the age of three. A trachy bypasses the vocal cords, so for her first three years, Emily had to be mute. She was an anxious and shy child, prone to cry in social situations – understandable if you're unable to express yourself verbally. Emily had to cry silently.

Beth had come out of hospital earlier; despite a diagnosis of cerebral palsy following her NICU haemorrhage, she was always the healthier one, and as a toddler she was vivacious, funny and cheeky. Allie and Tom knew she would always be physically disabled and would either use a wheelchair or be able to walk short distances. They expected she would attend mainstream school, then go to university.

Then, at the age of three, Beth started to have seizures. She developed two rare kinds of epilepsy which don't respond to treatment: Lennox Gastaut syndrome and another kind with the catchy title of constant spike wave of slow sleep. No one can be certain about the cause of Beth's epilepsy, but it's likely a delayed result of the haemorrhage she suffered in the neo-natal unit.

At the age of six, when I first met the family, Beth was having seizures every few minutes, all the time. Unable to sleep normally, her development had regressed. When Joel and I visited one summer afternoon, Beth was able to crawl in the garden, wearing a helmet to protect her head from knocks when she had seizures, but was unable to speak or sign. Her gaze moved towards familiar people and she liked listening to stories, but there was no way of knowing whether she grasped what was said around her. Allie and Tom believed she could not understand abstract concepts and considered her mental age that of a baby. Beth did not know the difference between day and night, for instance, and so Allie and Tom took turns to sleep next to her and try to settle her through each night.

Emily's life also changed when she was three, but for the better. She had gradually been weaned off the oxygen and was breathing air, so the trachy came out. Still, after the initial excitement of Emily talking for the first time, it began to be clear that she had difficulty communicating. When she started school, the intensely quiet and shy girl with light brown hair struggled to socialize. Her sensitivity to noisy environments meant the family couldn't take her into a cafe without her screaming. Like Joel, Emily would often put her hands over her ears, finding loud or unexpected sounds frightening, even painful. When Joel and I first visited, Emily hid in her room, polite but silent. Her physical coordination was also awkward. At six she was diagnosed with autism and, despite being an intelligent girl who could write, considerable learning difficulties. She was managing at mainstream school with one-to-one support, though she wasn't asked to many playdates, while Beth went to a special school. Both the twins were, at six, unable to eat orally and were fed entirely by gastrostomy. Between them they had undergone more than ten operations in the first years of their lives.

Joel and I visited again when the twins were seven. Beth lay in a big blue playpen with soft sides, Allie occasionally lifting and repositioning her. Emily smiled shyly through her pink glasses at Joel and me and brought us a pile of her favourite Charlie and Lola books to see. She was still quiet, but had such an intelligent and sweet presence, and I thought she and Joel seemed happy to play alongside each other, reassured by each other that they weren't the only one to find some things in life difficult. Emily vanished, and I heard someone on the piano playing 'I Hear Thunder' with great proficiency. I assumed it must be Tom, but it was in fact Emily. She had taught herself to play it.

Emily had achieved so much, yet the impact of her first ten months in hospital cannot be overestimated. As Allie outlined it to me in her honest way: 'When you think what other ten-month-olds' lives are like, they've had nothing but what you hope for your child – love, nurturing, fun, giggles, laughs – well, these children haven't. They've had pain, they've had threatening adults come up and say, "Hi Emily, don't worry, it's going to be fine," and then they jab you and they hurt you and they say, "Don't worry, you're being so brave." No wonder these kids have attachment disorders.'

It would be fairly miraculous for a child to develop neuro-logically normally in that situation, I said, and Allie agreed. One thing she'll never forget is the first day she took Emily out of the hospital in a buggy, just for half an hour, at eight and a half months old. Emily sat with her head nestled into the side of the buggy the entire time. She didn't know to look around, because she'd never been outside.

Allie, a serious woman, the kind who has a few close friend-ships rather than many superficial ones, still hasn't processed how traumatic her own experience as a mother has been; talk-ing to me about it was unusual for her. Old friends, she told me, 'want everything to be OK, they try and look for the posi-tives: "She's doing so well, you're so amazing, I don't know how you do it." Well, I'm not some magic woman; I'm some-one this happened to.' She had to work to initiate playdates for Emily, and then the difference between Emily and the other child would be so painful that often it felt easier not to arrange another playdate.

Like me, Allie has plagued herself with guilt. 'I could have done loads more for my kids. When your child has disabilities and special needs, nothing comes naturally. Your child's development doesn't just happen. Rolling over, sitting up, speaking, how to relate to other children, everything. Pushing up on the tummy was a massive undertaking with a blooming physiotherapist to tell you how to do it, and you had to prac-tise, and if you didn't practise you were failing your child. When the responsibility is the parent's, suddenly all these sup-posedly natural things become your responsibility as a mother, and that's a massive burden.'

The older disabled babies get, the more different they can seem from their peers. Take Leo, the mute but highly affec-tionate son of a friend of mine. When he first met Joel, the two of them – both innocents – immediately gave each other an enormous hug. Leo has a rare chromosomal microduplication and developmental delays, low muscle tone and motor skills problems. Aged six, Leo was in mainstream school, in a year group with boys who played football and chess, and were read-ing Harry Potter. Leo was still toilet training. He couldn't or wouldn't poo on the toilet. While a typical child may pick skills up by watching and modelling what others do – deciding to use the toilet, sitting and wiping, for instance – none of this was obvious for Leo. And his incontinence meant he couldn't easily attend mainstream holiday clubs; going out as a family often involved scrabbling around on the floor in a public toilet while Leo panicked at the sound of the hand dryer.

Although not clearly autistic, Leo has certain traits, like an obsession with washing machines – their noise, their spinning, the numbers on the dial – which has grown and grown. He excitedly shows his mother Kira pictures of washing machines in catalogues or in the house photographs in estate agent windows. The first thing he does on entering someone's home is find their washing machine. If Kira doesn't get to him in time, he will put a load of washing on and change the settings. 'Can't you just tell him not to?' a relative once asked Kira. 'You can't discipline this,' Kira replied. 'This is a force bigger than me.'

The other children at school 'definitely see him as different but not in a negative way thus far,' Kira told me. 'Which is lovely, but the cynic in me is like, when's it going to end? He needs so much more time for everything than everyone else.'

When people think of a child with a disability, they often think of autism, or wheelchairs, or Down's syndrome, or blindness. But outside the well-known categories, on the margins, are more and more children like Leo, Noah, Emily – or Joel – with barely understood special needs, whether genetic or those of the NICU veteran. They may not have clear-cut autism, for instance, but rather, autistic traits. They can run, but they are weak and tire easily. It's a mysterious and sometimes isolating, alienated margin to live in.

For Sophie, the doctor whose son Michael had fetal surgery for congenital diaphragmatic hernia, followed by six months in the neonatal unit after his birth at thirty-four weeks, life 'afterwards' has also not been easy.

Baby Michael had already had four general anaesthetics and four operations before he was born at thirty-three weeks. Michael was in neonatal intensive care for two months. A week after his birth, he had a six-hour surgery to fix the hernia. Two months after his birth, the diaphragm patch split. Michael had to undergo surgery again. Then, like Joel, he had a Nissen's fundoplication to control his reflux, but for Michael it was open surgery. Afterwards, his lung collapsed. They thought they were going to lose him. 'At that point I crumbled,' Sophie told me in her soft voice. She was referred for psychotherapy. 'I just couldn't take any more.'

When I visited them at home in a leafy English village when Michael was three, the handsome little chap was simultaneously watching *Paw Patrol*, jumping from chair to sofa and racing monster trucks – while maintaining an in-depth conversation about tyres. He was as lively as any other small boy, but he was attached to an oxygen tank so he could breathe. The long tube got wrapped around furniture when Michael jumped around and danced through the house, and Sophie, with her long wavy hair, jogged behind him, untying the knots it got into. Michael needed more oxygen at night and Sophie often slept in a bed in his room. When he went out, the adult with him wore a small oxygen tank on their back. Sophie was worried about his ability to join in at preschool with his one-to-one keyworker – the oxygen was so visible, and how would he keep up with the other children who could run unimpeded? Michael was also still mostly gastrostomy-dependent at three, unable to drink from an open cup and only eating a small amount, mainly toast.

Michael's lungs, stunted in utero, should grow, Sophie knew, and he was weaning off the oxygen. But the balloon procedure done when he was still unborn seemed to have had a long-term impact on his lungs – the cartilage in the big airways was soft and collapsed down, making his breathing harder. Michael had returned to hospital many times after picking up viruses. He had a chest deformity, chronic lung disease, severe reflux and developmental delay, and, when I met him, was still seeing ten specialists at different hospitals. Managing the appointments and staying on top of his health was a job in itself for Sophie, who was only able to return to her career as a hospital doctor two days a week with a lot of help from carers and grandparents.

From her dignified, calm appearance, I would never have guessed that Sophie believed she had PTSD. 'I've got massive ongoing issues,' she confessed in a fleeting quiet moment as we sat on her living room carpet. The fear was that each infection would take Michael back to intensive care or high dependency. 'I'm terrified of kids with snotty noses,' she told me. For ages she wouldn't take Michael anywhere; she avoided public places; there were no holidays. Even asymptomatic adults worried her. The sheer organization involved in travelling with the oxygen seemed too much, combined with the prospect of him getting unwell and not being near the local hospital, who know him. She would like counselling, she said to me, but didn't have time.

PTSD in parents who have 'done time' in the fetal or neonatal units is increasingly recognized, neonatal unit psychologist Rebecca Chilvers told me. More than 60 per cent of parents have an acute stress reaction to this situation, she estimated, which is sometimes the precursor to PTSD, which can improve, or not, over time. After leaving hospital, she says, some parents find intrusive thoughts about things they've seen or experienced coming to mind. 'That might be seeing their baby not breathing when they were born, it might be the panic alarm that sounds, it might be watching them put a tube in, or the moment that they realized everything was going wrong on delivery. They often have nightmares about it – people will wake up in the night and be very frightened as these things come back to them.'

Chilvers has seen parents of ten- or twelve-year-olds in tears talking about their neonatal experience a decade later. 'Parents are very isolated when they go home – going to mother-and-baby groups feels very different. Parents will say: "I tried to explain to people but they don't understand what it was like."'

As for having a child go through fetal surgery, fetal neuro-surgeon Greg Heuer at CHOP remarked to me: 'It's not unlike a child who survives cancer. It changes life forever. These kids tend to be more spoiled. They're special, in a good way.' The parents of fetal medicine survivors, he told me, 'are really attuned to their kids, for the rest of their lives'. He comforts mothers: 'You can prove you love your child like nobody else can because of what you went through.'

*

I wish I could have known in the dark days that everything was going to turn out so well for Joel. That the diagnosis didn't mean that the frightening things the doctors mentioned or that I Googled would happen. People with Noonan's are often late bloomers. Joel not only survived but his heart settled. He was able to breathe. He could eat, drink and digest without tubes. He no longer needed much medication, then none at all. The pain and discomfort he suffered in his first and second years disappeared completely. He blossomed into a funny, creative, loving (and good-looking) boy who other children and adults alike think is super-cool. After that sports day when all the older children at school cheered his name, I asked his teacher how all these kids even knew Joel. 'Oh, but Joel's *really* popular,' she said, surprised I hadn't realized. 'It's because he's so friendly.' Joel lives with an intensity and sensitivity unlike any one I have ever known. He likes to dress up in a crocodile suit and jump into ball pits; he makes vivariums in his bedroom filled with leaves and pebbles from the garden for his toy reptiles; he is a gifted artist who can turn junk into a 3D bat or Venus flytrap.

I wish I could have known Joel would be so happy and strong, and life would become good again. Instead of a baby who died in the womb or at birth, I was presented with my extraordinarily caring boy whose fascinations have ranged from Concorde to scary animals, but who steadfastly adores sausages.

We have been stupendously fortunate, I now know. I've seen how extreme prematurity can in itself cause disability as premature babies grow up. I think of the mothers whose babies didn't survive. I meet other children who have needs far more complex than Joel's – children who can't communicate; children who will never be able to live independent lives; children who will be tube-fed and on oxygen indefinitely; children who will never be able to sit or walk; children who live more or less in hospital; children who won't make it past adolescence.

These days, medicine keeps alive infants who would previously have died, but some of these children have congenital disorders that can't yet be cured. Their lives are lived largely in hospital, hooked up to life-support machines. It's another 'grey area' created by medicine pushing back the limits of life and death; what the pioneering children's surgeon Everett Koop called 'the double-edged sword of modern medicine, the ability of high-tech medicine to extend human life, for better or for worse'.[14] At birth, it's often impossible to predict whether a child will end up having a chance of a good quality of life, beyond intensive care. Children live, but then sometimes, after a period of months or years, parents and doctors have to make an impossible choice about what makes a child's life worth living. Anyone who has seen a child wide awake on a ventilator, trying to tear it out of their throat because it's so oppressive and uncomfortable, anyone who has seen a child's eyes roll back as the morphine sedates them, or who has seen a child wail in pain at being covered in catheters knows that a life of intensive care interventions with no end in sight is full of suffering. But is it kinder to let that suffering end, or to continue with a very difficult life?

In 2004, newborn Daisy Nimmo, the fourth child of Stephanie, a marketing consultant, and Andy, a corporate trainer, became one of the first children to be diagnosed with the gene for Costello syndrome – a rasopathy like Noonan's, but far rarer and considered more severe. Modern medicine made Daisy's life possible, but she spent much of it in hospital suffering from multiple chronic conditions. 'You become a prisoner – you're in a goldfish bowl,' Stephanie told me of her family's years in hospital wards.

Somehow, in spite of being one of the sickest children the nurses at Great Ormond Street had ever seen, Daisy often seemed 'as strong as an ox, so incredibly full of life and happy'. But the family realized that Daisy couldn't keep bouncing back forever. There would be a crisis, at some point.

At the age of eleven, Daisy's body became colonized by sepsis, infections caused by 'so much plastic in her': a central

line, a gastrostomy which drained bile from her stomach, an
ileostomy and stoma bag, a stoma in the bladder. The bugs
clung hard to the plastic and Daisy had developed antibiotic
resistance.

'People are scared of death,' Stephanie said to me. 'They're
scared of not doing enough for their child, but actually sometimes doing enough for your child is letting them go and
letting them die.' When septic shock took over and Daisy's
tiny body slowed down, in January 2017, that time did come.

In intensive care, one day, Daisy had a cardiac arrest. Stephanie walked into the ward to find doctors resuscitating her. 'I
didn't want her to die,' she told me. But she said to the doctors: 'If she goes, then let her go.' To bring her back would just
be delaying the inevitable.

Stephanie asked the hospital if Daisy could die at home.
But the hospital said she was too unstable to leave; she might
end up having a cardiac arrest and dying in an ambulance in
central London.

So they let her go there, in the children's hospital, the life-
support machine turned off, holding her hands as she took her
last breath. Daisy had spent twelve years in this world.

'I don't use euphemisms like "passed away",' Stephanie told
me. 'What am I doing? Am I protecting you? She died. It's
horrible, it cuts you, that's reality.' Phrases like dead children
'gaining their wings', she said, 'wouldn't wash with my boys.
She's died. Her energy has just gone out. That's it. Death is
the end.'

And yet . . . 'We need to find meaning out of what has happened.' Stephanie – an energetic woman, the kind who runs
marathons – was driven to find meaning by doing good after
her family's unimaginable loss. Having considered training as

a nurse, she has written a blog and books about Daisy[15] and educates healthcare workers on how to support families.

Many of the people I spoke to when writing this book have redirected their lives in the light of their experiences. NICU mother Eve shifted from occupational therapy to family therapy, writing her thesis on the psychological effect of premature birth on parents. Hayley Goleniowska and Caroline White started blogs about Down's syndrome. Judith Van de Meerakker was inspired by her heart condition to get a PhD in the genetics of heart defects. Jess has raised money for the fetal medicine unit where she lost her son Corey in an EXIT procedure. When I interviewed Jess, she told me she was planning to visit the fetal medicine unit again: 'I've been thinking about them a lot recently. I feel connected to them.' Sophie is still in touch with the doctor who first resuscitated Michael and another who saved his life several times in the neonatal unit. I wrote this book and – without any conscious intention – I have also found myself making friends with the parents at Joel's school who are doctors. I know they will understand what Joel and my family have been through.

'You almost *become* a doctor in a way,' Allie once reflected to me of her neonatal experience. 'The people who are relating to your child aren't cousins, aunts, uncles, best friends – they're doctors; nurses.' The doctors and nurses in the unit become like the child's family, they are the people who shared the child's first months and got to know their character before extended families and friends. No wonder the bond with these people becomes so important for parents – and, sometimes, in time, the grown-up children. A few years ago, Charles, one of the first people to undergo fetoscopy, in 1983, visited his namesake Charles Rodeck, bearing gifts of an Australian bush hat and some pipe tobacco – his parents had told him about

Rodeck's one-time habit, now long since given up. The young man seemed surprised at first to see that this man, whom he had imagined as a godlike giant, was so short. But Rodeck, he found, was just as kind and compassionate as he had always believed. It meant a great deal to young Charles to meet the man who saved his life and go out to dinner together. And for Rodeck, seeing this man, of whom his last memory was a sick baby, was 'extraordinary'. He felt humbled.

*

Every year since 1996, CHOP has held a reunion for the children who were treated there as fetuses. The first party, in 1996, had ten families attending. By the time I attended one in 2018, there were 400 families from twenty-six states; Hawaii to Florida to Maine. The attendees ranged in age from twenty-three to in utero, but most were pre-teens.

In typical CHOP style, this was a celebration to the max, like nothing any NHS hospital would think up. Beach towels and T-shirts were given away with slogans: 'We dare to dream!' and 'Dreams do come true!' Every child was given a name sticker colour-coded for the condition she or he had been treated for – red and black for CHAOS syndrome, blue for lung lesions, black for sacrococcygeal teratoma – so they could network. Families lined up to chat with Scott Adzick, dressed down in casual slacks and a denim shirt, who confessed to me, 'It's a little overwhelming.' It's the doctors' favourite day of the year, but as overjoyed as they are to see the fruits of their labours, they also think about the children who aren't here – the cases that didn't work out.[16]

A lot of families make the reunion part of their summer vacation. Easy listening jazz played as everyone gathered in a marquee on the hospital grounds, grazing on a huge buffet. It seemed a matter of pride to the families to be here, part of an exclusive club. Parents wore their own T-shirts proclaiming 'Mama bear', 'CDH warrior', 'I have a hero: I call her my daughter'. TV and radio stations were filming and interviewing. The crowd was given a hashtag for their social media posting about today's event: #CHOPfetalreunion. Philly police officers, with shiny belts and badges, and rifles and pistols, lined up as the children went on stage to sing the national anthem and pledge allegiance to the flag. Then, they marched on stage military-style. ('Mom, why do they have guns?' one little boy sitting behind me asked.) Later there would be candyfloss and cupcakes, face painting, bouncy castles, a climbing wall, a carousel and slides.

I spoke to fifteen-year-old Connor, one of the first to have spina bifida surgery in utero here, and his mother Pegeen, a piano teacher, father Frank, a media consultant, and older brother Ryan. Pegeen was still wiping her eyes after hearing her baby had spina bifida when she was offered the referral for experimental surgery at CHOP. The local hospital where she got the diagnosis had told her, 'You might not want to have this baby.' She would have had him no matter what, she told me, but the surgery at CHOP had given her an option mothers didn't have before. Apart from a slightly different gait and minor balance problems, Connor has grown up strong and healthy, and these days, Dr Adzick was thrilled to hear, he's into tap dancing.

The hospital chaplain gave a speech. 'Some miracles come into being in the most challenging of ways,' she said, asking God's blessing as we do the 'unimaginable'. Next, everyone watched a video on a big screen which showed photographs of each child survivor holding a sign saying what they wanted to do or be when they grew up: 'a veterinarian', 'to be kind', 'to live, John 3:16', 'to have my own pony', 'a baseball player', 'a farmer', 'a giraffe' (the crowd laughed) – and a great number of wannabe doctors and nurses.

'Whatever struggles they have, they've been through worse,' the voiceover proclaimed. 'Yes, you can cry.' So many previously unliveable lives were going to be lived, and with so much hope and happiness. I didn't want to cry because a video had made me, but tears came and I wept along with everyone else.

*

How did Joel's life turn out? That is his story, not mine.

All I can say is this.

Was our family life 'normal'? Not exactly. It probably never would have been, though.

Did Joel continue to need specialist doctors and nurses? Yes.

Was life easy? Not always.

Was it boring? Never.

Was Joel happy? Yes.

Was I happy? Yes.

10

Knowing

Joel lived. We loved him more than anything in the world and our family life was happy in his third year. Phil and I had always wanted two children and now that Joel was no longer ill, the time seemed right to try again. And this time, before we even conceived, we had to work out how much we wanted to know.

We hoped our next baby would not have health or developmental problems. I would not wish illness for any baby, and the idea of going through what Joel had in hospital again was frightening. We also worried it would be unfair for Joel to have a sibling with as many additional needs as he had. I had long since embraced my child's differences – but although I felt guilty for thinking it, the idea of bringing up *two* children with extra needs was daunting. Then again, perhaps I could embrace that too, as many parents do.

On a less rational level, it seemed almost impossible to me that we could have a healthy baby. I still had a fear from my pregnancy with Joel – that there was something wrong with me and that I would have one sick baby after another. But our clinical geneticist was clear: because Joel's Noonan syndrome was 'de novo' – not inherited – our chance of another baby with the same condition was less than 1 per cent. This was slightly higher than someone in the general population, because it was possible that although Phil and I do not have Noonan's, some of my egg cells or Phil's sperm cells might have it and others not: an untestable, 'mosaic' version of Noonan syndrome.

The only way for us to know at the start of a pregnancy whether the embryo had Noonan's would be to have pre-implantation genetic diagnosis – a procedure developed in the early 1990s. It's much like IVF – eggs are fertilized and embryos tested in the lab for 'defects' before a healthy one is placed in the womb – but the geneticist told us that our chance of another baby with Noonan's was far too low to warrant this. There were a few options, she said. We could go through the pregnancy with the usual screening, plus extra ultrasound scans, which would either reassure us or give some indication if something was not normal, but we wouldn't know for certain until the baby was born whether it had Noonan's. Today, I might have had a non-invasive NIPT blood test which claims to tell with more than 99 per cent certainty whether a baby has Noonan's or not,[1] but it wasn't available in 2013. At the time, we could have a CVS or amniocentesis, which could tell us if the baby had Noonan's. Phil and I didn't want to do this – we weren't willing to risk the small chance of miscarriage after an invasive test.

We'll cross an ethical quagmire if we come to it, Phil and I decided. In the end, pregnancy is a game of chance.

Because of our previous high-risk pregnancy with Joel, when we did conceive again, the fetal medicine doctors at UCH gave us several early scans simply for reassurance. There was no bleeding and all appeared normal, but by the time of the nuchal translucency scan, my teeth were starting to chatter again.

This time the nuchal screen was over quickly, with a measurement so low, so far from any border, that there could be no cause for worry. My 'risk' of a baby with a chromosomal condition was one in tens of thousands, not hundreds. How random these all-important numbers still appeared – almost nothing to do with a baby, just a good or bad number thrown down from on high. More scans followed, every couple of weeks. An early, detailed anomaly scan at seventeen weeks with a consultant, and a heart scan, were the next hurdles; they would be hunting for any sign, however small, of anything abnormal. Surely, I thought, they would spot some problem.

But they couldn't find anything wrong. In the photo Phil and I took of ourselves on a bench in Bloomsbury, immediately after we left the fetal medicine unit clutching the scrap of notepaper on which the scanner had penned in curly handwriting the word 'female', there's a glimmer of peace in my eyes.

The months rolled on smoothly, but then at twenty-eight weeks, my mind started to turn to how, at this stage in my pregnancy with Joel, everything had gone wrong.

When I felt some strange tightening sensations, I assumed they must be Braxton Hicks practice contractions, but called the midwife. What happened next was eerily familiar from the day before Joel was born premature.

I was sent to UCH. A midwife hooked me up to a machine to check for contractions. Around midnight, a doctor, a junior one, came. She said the monitor showed I had had a few small contractions. I asked if they could be Braxton Hicks. She wasn't sure. She said she was going to examine me and give me a fibronectin test and offered to explain. But since this was exactly what happened a few hours before Joel was born, it was already clear in my memory – a vaginal swab that could indicate if I was in premature labour, or likely to go into it. The results would be back in seven minutes, she said. Phil, at home with Joel, was waiting anxiously for them too.

Left alone in the examination room for an hour, I waited but no one came. Finally I went to find the midwife, who said my case was being discussed with a senior doctor. My heart sank; this didn't sound good.

Then the midwife came in and said: 'We're going to admit you. The test came back positive. You have to have steroids now.'

I burst into tears and said, 'I can't do this again. This can't be happening again.' I could be in premature labour – and this time at twenty-eight weeks. I lay on my own on the couch, crying, for fifteen minutes.

Back on the bustling ward where I'd been the night before giving birth to Joel, in a bed next to two mothers with crying newborn babies, at 1.30 a.m. I had the steroid injection, and a sleepless night. History seemed to be repeating itself. But the next day, it was decided that I was not in labour and that I just had an infection, for which I needed antibiotics. A scan confirmed that there was no hydrops. The baby was fine. After a second round of steroids I was allowed home, sure everything now would be well. The milestone of thirty-two weeks came and went uneventfully.

The day I hit thirty-five weeks was a Monday morning. For a few days I'd felt stomach cramps like period pains; the hospital had checked me out and they had sent me home. This time, though, the feelings were stronger. And then my waters broke.

Within ten minutes Phil and I were in a taxi. That journey

into central London with the pain ratcheting itself up with each contraction, now only two minutes apart, seemed long. Although I wasn't too worried about our baby because thirty-five weeks is barely premature, I prayed she was not going to need the neonatal care unit.

The last time I'd seen the glamorous and charming Colombian neonatal consultant Angela Huertas-Ceballos, she'd been at one of Joel's heart scans in the neonatal unit when he had just been saved from heart failure. It was surreal to see her again, in the labour suite. She told me our daughter was going to be fine. The doctors didn't know why she was early but suspected it might be because I'd had a virus with a high fever the previous week.

Just before I gave birth after nine hours of labour, Judith Meek appeared by my side – the fairy godmother was there just in time, as ever.

Our little girl Anna had curly red hair. She cried right away. She could breathe perfectly and was a healthy size and colour. She was brought to my arms and immediately began breast-feeding. I lay on the hospital bed in near silence in the night just gazing at her happily for many hours. I thought: 'This baby is going to have a wonderful life.'

Anna was very healthy for thirty-five weeks, but she was small – less than 5 lbs – and some jaundice developed, so we were kept in hospital for eight days. Thankfully, Anna was nursed in an open cot next to me on the postnatal ward – no special care unit or incubator for her.

That short week brought back memories of what we'd been through with Joel. Anna had a cannula put in her hand and was sleeping under a special jaundice light. It didn't help that I hadn't been outside the hospital ward in days, but in my postnatal haze, I was in floods of tears – which made me realize how strong I'd had to be for Joel, who had been through a thousand times worse. Because I hadn't been able to stay with him or breastfeed him, and he'd been in an incubator attached to so many tubes, and it hadn't been safe enough for me to hold him for the first days of his life, I'd seen everything done to him at a sort of remove.

Now, with Anna, I was with her like a normal mother – 24/7 – and I had to see every needle put in her and hold her little body glowing with a light pad to help clear her jaundice. She wasn't actually terribly bothered by these small medical interventions – she was quite an easy-going baby – but I wept more for what Joel had been through than what Anna was experiencing. In his case, he'd had jaundice but we'd barely registered it, because it was the least of his medical problems.

I felt silly thinking about the past in this way. Phil kept saying, 'But look at Joel now; that's all behind us – and Anna is doing so well.' There was someone else I needed. I called in my friend Eve, Noah's mother. When she walked into my cubicle with a bag full of premature baby clothes for me (we had long since given Joel's old ones away as I could not bear the sight of them), I knew it could not be easy for her to return to a maternity ward.

'Is this hard for you?' I asked Eve.

'Just going up in a hospital lift still sends shivers of dread through me,' she confessed.

I knew the feeling. It was so brave and kind of her to come despite this, and her presence that day gave me the strength I needed to relax and enjoy my essentially well baby. Soon we were out of hospital and I re-donated those premature baby clothes to the neonatal unit.

From the start, Anna was different from Joel. She held her head up strongly from early on, she drank easily and often, and she happily lay on her stomach and tried to roll. I only had to look at her bonny little thighs to know how healthy she was (Joel's have always been stick-like, no matter how much he eats). She seemed textbook normal.

Even so, at the back of my mind there was still a belief that Anna might turn out have Noonan's, or some disease, yet to be diagnosed. My experience with Joel had left me with a continuing fear that the shockingly unexpected could and would happen; that maybe I couldn't have healthy babies. So I booked an appointment with Joel's clinical geneticist at Great Ormond Street.

I was expecting the geneticist to take blood from Anna to send to the lab. I would have welcomed such watertight confirmation that she was 'fine', simply to put my mind at rest – though I also worried that the result might find some other thing wrong we hadn't even considered. But instead, examining my daughter, she pronounced her so clearly normal that blood testing was absolutely uncalled for.

I struggled to take in those words. How could she be so confident, especially when Joel, to me, looked normal too? But she insisted that all the signs were that this baby was fine. And then she said: 'Actually Joel's ears are rather low-set. But perhaps I'm being unfair.'

She said, 'Anna is beautiful.'

I couldn't help thinking: 'Would you not say that if she had signs of the syndrome? Isn't my son beautiful too?'

And then I thought how hard it must be to do the job of a clinical geneticist diagnosing babies. How every word you say can mean so much to a parent.

Although Anna was technically premature, at thirty-five weeks exactly, I have never thought of her as a prem-born child, and never been very concerned about any impact of prematurity on her development. There was too much of a universe of difference between her week of recovery from jaundice by my side in the postnatal ward and all that Joel went through.

As Anna grew up, with no health problems, things came instinctively to her: at five months she was holding her own bottle to feed herself, examining baby toys with interest, loved walks in the woods – she could handle the bumpy ride because she was mesmerized by the leaves in the trees. And she easily took to all kinds of music, pictures, sensations and play, sitting quiet and smiling on my lap. The way she learned was exponential, automatic. One new thing led organically to ten more: her mind leaped to grasp new connections and the gaps in between were filled in as if by magic. Having another, 'typical' child can be healing for a mother of a child born with a disability. It can also throw the other child's struggles into sharper relief. I now fully understood how much harder life was for Joel than for the average child. He was bright and curious but learned in a more linear way, painstakingly, nothing taken for granted. My son was needy, in his own world, didn't learn practical skills easily. Joel was the eternal innocent; he wished he didn't have to grow up, wanting to play forever. My daughter, by contrast, was strong, worldly and independent.

And lovely as it was to have an 'easy' baby as well, I also truly enjoyed the challenge that opening Joel's eyes to all the things in the world gave me as a mother; I appreciated the reward of his every achievement and happiness.

*

May 2017. I stood in a conference room in Sutton Coldfield surrounded by people with whom I had nothing in common other than the fact our children shared a genetic difference.

It's a bizarre way for people to come together. I wondered, when I planned to attend the UK Noonan Syndrome Association annual families' day for the first time, whether when Joel finally got to meet other people with Noonan syndrome he would feel some sort of recognition, feel somehow at home with them. It was a silly idea; I was wrong.

Six-year-old Joel proclaimed the entire get-together 'boring'. He did not recognize himself in the other children; did not want to make friends; did not particularly like anyone. He just wanted to go home.

It was the first time we had ever (knowingly) met anyone else with Noonan's. The children with my son's diagnosis were not carbon copies of one another. A few were in wheelchairs, while others stunned me by their agility playing ping-pong or rock climbing. Some looked noticeably tiny or different facially; others did not. They played excitedly and contentedly, and behaved beautifully – it was only my son who found the noise of the crowd unbearable and didn't want to join in. I realized then that any difficulties my son had might be less connected with his genetics and perhaps more with having spent so much of his first two years in hospital or in discomfort – on top of prematurity. The fact that our children were genetically similar meant I and the other parents could share stories of particular symptoms and experiences, but on another level, I discovered there was no deeper sense of finding one's genetic family.

How do you tell a child that he has a genetic difference? Phil and I thought a lot about when and how to give Joel this self-knowledge. It could be a shocking thing to discover about yourself – and yet more and more children are in the position of accepting such revelations. Some families of children with genetic conditions talk about the diagnosis with them and around them from babyhood to avoid any surprise; others decide to hold the information back until a certain point when the child can understand better what it means. Some adults with genetic conditions were not told about their diagnoses until they grew up, and sometimes this meant struggling for years wondering why they were different, without any answers. One woman with Noonan syndrome posted on Facebook: 'I just think telling them is important for them to have an understanding WHY. Why we are so small, why we have so many doctors to see, why we get sick and hurt easier than most, why we struggle to understand basic life skills and why we are "different".'

Phil and I decided to wait for Joel to notice he had some differences from others and to ask us about them. In his second year of school, he started to observe that he was smaller than others his age, and to ask why he fell over so often. He also knew, by then, about the fact that he had been very ill at the start of his life. That Christmas it seemed right to tell him about Noonan syndrome. How odd it felt to me to have known the words of this condition and to filter so much through the diagnosis for five years, but for my son not to have any knowledge of something which had played a significant part in his life and possibly always would. In the end we spent five minutes mentioning the words Noonan syndrome, telling Joel that he was built a bit differently and this was why he sometimes needed a bit of extra help. We told him that he was special and should be proud of all he had been through and achieved. Phil and I felt very serious; it was a big moment for us.

'OK,' said Joel, bored, and wandered off to play with his toy planes. Since then, when occasionally he has expressed a wish to be as tall and able to do things as easily as other children, it's been hard to know what to say. I want to be positive about it, to treat him like anyone else and never limit him, but also not to lie to Joel, to deny his struggle and say that it's insignificant to go through all he does. He refuses to be patronized. One morning when Joel was seven, on the way to one of his myriad hospital check-ups, he asked, 'Why do I have to do this all the time?' I'd been advised by other parents of disabled children to tell my son he was a 'superhero', so I tried it. 'But I don't want to be a silly superhero,' he retorted sadly. All I could do was reassure him again and again that he was special and that being different was OK. But why should he have to be a 'superhero' or a 'warrior' or any of the other clichés with which people talk about children with health problems?

The euphemistic assumptions people make about sickly infants are easy and almost automatic, much like the agreed cuteness of kittens and bunny rabbits. They are 'little fighters', 'miracles'. They supposedly 'fly high with the angels' when they die, leaving only sadface emojis behind. For me it has never been like this. I didn't believe in angels or miracles. My radiant son wasn't a brave little soldier; he was too pure and innocent to know what bravery or war were. The weaker babies who die, I knew, are no less brave than the ones who pull through. Speaking of bravery, doesn't that imply making a choice to face the worst? In that case, sick babies aren't especially brave and neither were Phil and I as parents. We lived through that experience because we had to. There was no other choice. The only bravery of the fetal and neonatal units is simply getting through each day.

It didn't occur to me at the time Joel was in hospital that anyone might feel for me as his mother. In the years that followed, when I told Joel's story to anyone, they typically said 'What a hard time you had' and I felt touched. There were people wanting to comfort me, full of love for us, during the five months Joel spent in the neonatal unit too, and in the weeks after his birth we were flooded with cards and gifts for him, but although I typed out thank yous on my phone while riding the underground into town to be with Joel each morning, I barely looked at the sweet sleepsuits and toys that friends and family sent. In his incubator Joel wore nothing but a micronappy provided by the hospital. The time when Joel would play with toys or be able to wear even clothes designed for prem babies seemed impossibly distant – and even if he could wear clothes, how would all the tubes keeping him alive and monitoring him fit around one of the cute sleepsuits without a front opening? It never crossed my mind to feel secure in a general feeling of sympathy, to be 'the poor mother with the ill baby' in the popular imagination.

Looking back, I could have felt sorry for myself, defined myself as 'the parent of the sick child', a type of virtue signalling. (Ian Brown, author of *The Boy in the Moon*, a memoir about his son with another rasopathy called CFC syndrome, describes 'disability masochists . . . who seemed to relish their hardship and the opportunity to make everyone else feel guilty and privileged . . . their sense of angry entitlement, their relentless self-pity masquerading as bravery and compassion . . .'[2]) Then no one is allowed to offend you or challenge you. You are always the one who has the privilege of victim status, to whom everyone must be kind. But when Joel was ill, I felt as far as you can get from that easy sympathetic world of hearts melting for sick and disabled kiddies.

There's something phoney in a response to a child's illness of gathering a sentimental but ignorant army, of refusing in extreme cases to let a terminally ill baby die, of against all odds insisting the parent knows better than any doctor. The only way forward when a baby is very ill is to get on with reality. As the journalist Zoë Williams once wrote, 'radical barbarism and self-sacrifice are almost never what's required when your child is in jeopardy in real life: rather, qualities that are so far out of reach that they are neither superhuman nor inhuman, simply impossible. The dispassionate acceptance of a reality that is unacceptable; the clear-sighted evaluation of a situation that cannot be borne.'[3]

Years later, when I spoke about disability with two friends who have physical disabilities (they jokingly call themselves 'crips', short for cripples), they told me that they shared my scepticism about ill baby clichés. They were furious about society's visible support for parents of sick children, but not for disabled people once they grow up. In their view, many parents of disabled children grabbed all the sympathy they could get and built their lives around being the parent of a disabled child and the validation, attention and support this brought them – the parent, in effect, gets all the 'nice' parts of disability without actually having to be the one with the disability.

It's hard not to accept attention and validation. Parents of disabled children are devoted, work hard and have difficult lives – they deserve support. But how easy it is to fall into the persona of the virtuous parent of a disabled child who is a 'little miracle'. And what will it be like for these 'little miracles' when they are middle-aged and not so cute anymore?

*

A smiling woman in a floral dress breezed me through a door marked with orange warning stickers: 'Biological Hazard'; 'TOXIC'. The Institute for Women's Health is a nondescript old building with frosted windows, down a secluded mews a couple of blocks from UCH. We walked through laboratories, and I was shown incubators full of cells infected with genetically modified viruses; a young female scientist was slicing dead mouse brains.

At the back of the lab was a deep freeze. Here lay samples from the placentas or blood of 110 women whose unborn babies had been diagnosed with fetal growth restriction (FGR), a condition affecting one in ten pregnancies, in which the baby's growth slows or even stops in utero. My tour guide in the flowery dress was the head of this lab, Professor Anna David, fetal medicine consultant at UCH, and head of its Prenatal Cell and Gene Therapy Group. She and her team, she explained, were using these samples to develop a test for a protein marker which will be able to predict whether a fetus at twenty weeks' gestation with FGR will continue to grow, or not. A baby that continues to grow can be delivered at around twenty-eight weeks, and survive, while other babies simply stop growing and die in utero before they reach that gestation.

In the near future, if a baby is found to have the marker which predicts a bad outcome, the mother will be eligible for gene therapy – one of the first trials of gene therapy on pregnant women, which Anna David is working on. The reason why babies stop growing properly in cases of FGR is because the mother's blood doesn't circulate to the uterus and placenta as well as it should. But injecting a genetically modified virus – of the kind we get when we have a cold – into the uterine arteries could increase the blood supply and make the baby grow again. Called a viral vector, this engineered virus is the ideal way to spread something quickly through local cells in the uterine circulation. The vector is modified to act only temporarily and so that it cannot replicate. After a week of producing the correct proteins to increase maternal blood flow, the blood supply to the womb is improved, and the viral vector is destroyed by the body. The technique is called maternal growth factor gene therapy.

Scientific advances now on the horizon will make much of the medical treatment described in this book, and practised currently, seem like the dark ages. Fetal and neonatal medicine have many 'fathers'; now it is the time for scientific 'mothers' of the field – like Anna David – to come forward.

Professor David had arrived to meet me right on time, yet full of apologies in her British way. She had come straight from seeing patients on the antenatal ward where I had gone into premature labour with Joel. 'Please don't apologize,' I said. 'I feel bad taking you away from your work.' There was friendliness and clarity in this woman's voice and shining from her eyes behind thick glasses. This specialist was not an intimidating god, but a down-to-earth human being. A mother of two teenage children, Anna lives in London, and loves gardening. 'I'm having great fun growing tomatoes,' she told me.

Thanks to researchers like Anna David, the fetal medicine unit will be a very different place by the time Joel grows up. Women are likely to have antenatal testing and treatment earlier, in the first months of pregnancy, and congenital anomalies that we currently think of as 'just one of those things' will likely turn out to have genetic explanations we can even treat. In the future, premature babies could be nursed not in incubators but in artificial wombs – an extraordinary idea researched by a brilliant CHOP scientist and surgeon called Alan Flake (who I was told was too shy to enjoy interviews).

In the last decade CHOP has started performing fetal cardiac surgery for the severe condition of hypoplastic left heart syndrome at twenty-six to twenty-eight weeks' gestation, when the heart is the size of a peanut. And if operating on a

peanut-sized heart sounds challenging, what about one the
size of a pea? Since the mid-1980s, fetal researchers have been
working on the possibility of stem cell transplants to treat diseases involving a single serious cell defect, like the red blood
cell disorders sickle-cell anaemia and thalassaemia, or immune
deficiency diseases like severe combined immunodeficiency
(SCID), a genetic disorder known as 'bubble boy disease' in
which children have very low resistance to infection and are
likely to die in infancy. Stem cells are a kind of superhero cell
the body makes which have the power to take on all kinds of
functions, from being an organ cell to a red blood cell or a
muscle cell, and can divide endlessly, renewing themselves
again and again to repair and replace faulty tissue. In 1996, a
still-experimental human fetal stem cell transplant saved the
life of an unborn baby. The mutation that causes SCID ran in
the family and had already killed the couple's first child. When
they became pregnant again, antenatal testing at twelve weeks
diagnosed this fetus with SCID. Alan Flake gave him a bone
marrow stem cell transplant in utero from his father, and the
boy grew up healthy.[4] A fetus has a relatively under-developed
immune system, so there's no need for immunosuppressant
drugs or fear of rejection, problems that affect transplantation
after birth.

Now, at CHOP, the team has developed a technique
through animal experimentation which will soon be able to
deliver stem cell transplants into the bottom left quarter of the
pea-sized hearts of twelve- to fourteen-week-old, thumb-sized
human fetuses with sickle-cell anaemia. The mother, whose
cells are healthy, will take medication to increase her produc-
tion of stem cells. The cells will be gathered through a needle
in the mother's vein, the cells isolated in a laboratory, and
then they will be injected under ultrasound guidance into the

perfect spot in the fetus's heart for the aorta to pump them around the body. Now the fetus will not only have their own sick cells but a small percentage of a healthy cell line, which, if given in time (sixteen weeks' gestation is too late) may multiply through the body and help halt the progression of the disease. After birth, a baby with this healthy cell line will then have an excellent chance of tolerating another bone marrow transplant without rejecting it.[5] The baby in utero will become what scientists call a 'chimera', named after the ancient Greek mythological creature, a hybrid of more than one animal.

Stem cell transplants are getting cleverer year by year – in 2019 we are seeing the first European clinical trials on human fetuses. Stem cells provide a new source of healthy cells to perform a function a fetus lacks, but they don't actually change the fetus's DNA. Altering fetal DNA – gene therapy – is still futuristic at this point, but it's coming. The viral vector Anna David is researching inserts itself only into the cytoplasm of the mother's cells – the part outside the nucleus – but other viral vectors could get into the nucleus and change chromosomes. Technically gene therapy could be given to the fetus directly to correct a genetic disease in the baby before birth – a controversial idea, because it would be hard to be confident of only reaching a given target. Altered gene coding could get into the fetus's germline in the ovaries or the testes, affecting future generations, or it could have 'off-target effects' on different organs. If we start targeting sickle cell or thalassaemia blood cells with gene therapy, for instance, we still aren't sure the gene wouldn't start targeting other tissues too. Also, the mother or fetus might have an immune reaction to the vector. Or the other genetic material in the virus (besides the genetically modified vector) could damage the fetus.

Further into the future will come gene editing, using CRISPR, a more targeted tool than gene therapy, which can cut out abnormal genes and replace them with normal ones. Being able to use CRISPR rather than viral vectors would allow us to avoid the risky side effects that might go with viral vectors. Its use in humans after birth – let alone before birth – is still years away but could be immensely powerful, able to cut out single-gene conditions like cystic fibrosis, or Noonan syndrome, not only in the affected fetus but in the DNA a fetus will pass on to their own children. For now, gene editing remains completely untested in human fetuses. The ethical issues of being able to eradicate genes permanently are highly sensitive. Gene editing could change a baby's hair colour – or IQ. Do we want a world without genetic mutation? This will be a question not for us but for Joel and his generation.

*

My son is well now, a hilarious and zany little schoolboy of eight, the shunt Peebles implanted still somewhere in his chest, causing no harm. One GOSH cardiothoracic surgeon told us he had only seen one other child with a shunt from fetal surgery inside them; this was barely performed before the mid-1990s, and even today, it's still uncommon. The consensus seems to be it's best to leave it in Joel's chest; cardiothoracic surgery isn't undertaken unless it's absolutely essential. Doctors are now having to explore new pathways for adults who were 'medical miracles' at birth, whose congenital defects, never previously treatable, have been fixed – but years later, after the child graduates from paediatric clinics, no one knows what monitoring and care they need. Complicated babies are becoming complicated children who become complicated adults.[6]

The hydrops became a memory; the two needle marks on either side of my belly disappeared within a couple of years; Joel's surgery scars still decorate his chest and abdomen but we no longer spend Saturday nights at A&E or have a special chest full of Joel's medicines. As Joel got better, I started using that bottle of perfume again; I lit the candles; I put threads in the sewing box; I got a new handbag; I went back to work; we had Anna.

I still don't know what Noonan syndrome means and neither does Joel. No one really does. It means different things to everyone who has it. It's impossible, if Joel behaves in any way unusually, to know if it's the syndrome, the prematurity, the long-term effects of spending his first five months in hospital and his first two years in discomfort, or all of these – or maybe it's 'just him'. As one adult with Noonan's wrote on Facebook, 'some days it plays a big part; sometimes not'.

But I hope that having lived past his early challenges, Joel's diagnosis will be just a health issue to monitor. I'm not sure whether he will feel his start in life significant. But it's the sort of experience a mother or father never gets over, and the way Joel's life began will never leave me.

Baby doctors have to weigh up terrible risks. They cannot become too emotionally involved; they have to see babies in utero less as individual boys and girls and more as cases – while to the mother, who can feel the baby moving and loves it so much, this is deeply personal. Sometimes, though, a bridge of understanding emerges between the doctor and the patient – when the mother goes back to the doctor with her now-healthy child and says: 'Look – this is what you did. This is the person you helped create.' And the doctor looks into that child's eyes.

Joel, who so easily might never have lived, has a fear of death unusual among children. 'I nearly died,' he said, when he was seven, sitting on my bed before school one morning. 'What if I had died?' he asked me, trying to grasp the immensity of this idea.

The older Joel grew, the more I realized just how dearly he loved life. That tough, grown-up element many children have, that instinctive protective armour which makes them seem jaded before their time, my Peter Pan boy doesn't have. He is utterly enthusiastic about the world (although he tells me he doesn't think he likes homework), endlessly curious and passionate for information, about everything from poisonous tree frogs to trapdoors to the universe. He is true of heart, and his heart is wide open, offered to anyone despite the vulnerability of feeling with acute sensitivity. Like a puppy, he never sulks or holds a grudge – snap at him and he wants to cuddle in return. He is unself-conscious and doesn't particularly notice what anyone else thinks. Joel's world is a world all of its own. When I send him to his room to get a pair of socks, he meanders down twenty minutes later with a toy snake. The bright, spindly-legged boy only outgrew his last pair of age 9–12 month shorts aged seven, but he's too busy running around pretending to be a wolf or hunting for mushrooms in the long grass to care. Last month, when a child asked him about his size, he proudly explained: 'I have Noonan syndrome. And I'm a wild puppy who loves jumping in puddles.'

Six years after Joel left hospital, we had one of our long talks as he lay in his red car bed, ready to fall asleep. Joel, we talked about so many things. We talked about dreams and you said you wanted us to find each other that night in our dreams. You asked why we need to dream. When I told you it's to process our days, you asked why dreams are then not realistic. I explained they are about feelings and we imagine things symbolizing our feelings. You then wondered if you were in fact dreaming as we spoke. I mentioned the difference between fantasy and reality and suggested you might become a writer as you have such a great imagination. No, you said, I don't want to be a writer. You said, what will you be when you grow up? I said I am grown-up and I am a writer. You said no, you're a mummy. You said you want to be a daddy and a headteacher when you grow up. And as a daddy you will make nice breakfasts.

You wanted to know about how long it would take to walk to Australia, and what electricity pylons are for. We talked about yesterday being the past and tomorrow being the future. I told you how people used to live without electricity for thousands of years and how we can't imagine what will happen in the future. You said you hoped people wouldn't have guns in future. I said once something's been invented it can't be uninvented and you said you wished people would forget guns.

You wanted to know if I loved you infinitely, and what would happen if you added another infinity on to infinity. You told me you were just a tiny newborn puppy wolf cub and so so tiny and so new. You said you had just arrived from the dog sanctuary on my doorstep in a cage, with a label on which it said your name was Popsy. You had thought no one wanted you in the sanctuary and now Daddy and I had chosen you and brought you to our house. You said you were very shy at first and then excited and would start jumping up and hugging us. I've only just arrived, you said. You're so scared of everything and everything is new. I think that is how you feel a lot of the time – like a vulnerable new baby in need of protection.

I am honoured to know you and be your mother. You are an artist, an explorer, a philosopher and a poet, a liver of life, a lover of life. A remarkable person, deeply full of love and inquiry. Your final question as I left you to fall asleep was how long would it take to walk from England to the infinite? Forever, I said.

*

These days, Joel is keen to revisit the hospital where his life was saved, and we will soon set off to tread those lonely corridors again, together, his love giving me the strength I didn't have when he was a baby.

'Did the doctors love me?' he asks.

'Yes,' I say. 'Yes they did.'

At the Time of Writing . . .

Maeve, who was operated on in utero for sacrococcygeal teratoma, is meeting all milestones. She loves her big brothers, shoes and running around outside. 'She is feisty (as she has been since in utero), sassy and funny – full of life and love,' says her mother Kelly.

Michael, who had fetal surgery for congenital diaphragmatic hernia, settled into his first year at school part-time well and is making friends. He's crazy about space and can name all the planets in the solar system in order – including the dwarf planets. His mother Sophie hopes he will be free of his oxygen tank within the next year. She still hasn't had time for counselling.

Jess and Will started to try to conceive again a few months after Corey's death following a fetal EXIT procedure. Jess feared people would think she was 'such an awful mother – that I didn't care about Corey any more'. But having another child was a way forward. Their son, Lucas, was born big and healthy. When people ask, 'Is this your first child?' Jess replies, 'No, my first passed away.' They recently fell pregnant a third time.

Charles, the boy from the remote Australian town who was one of the first to undergo fetoscopy, is now in his thirties and works as an entertainer at a theme park, his only health trouble asthma. He and his wife recently had their first baby.

Noah, born at twenty-three weeks, is, aged eight, never happier than when pretending to play his guitar while listening to what he calls 'a heavy beat' on the radio. He is going to be a rock star.

Beth, born at twenty-five weeks, recently amazed everyone by identifying people from a choice of two photographs, showing that she knows the names of all the pupils and teachers in her class at school.

Emily, born at twenty-five weeks, is working hard on juggling and hula hooping. She can recite entire Charlie and Lola stories from memory and plays 'I Hear Thunder' on the piano a lot, every day.

Seb, who has Down's syndrome, eats, sleeps and breathes football. 'We were incredibly proud to see him play in several matches in his mainstream school's A Team this year,' his mother Caroline says. Seb models, recently for Marks and Spencer.

Natty, who has Down's syndrome, loves swimming, dancing and performing, cooking together with her mother Hayley, and learning how to buy things herself in the supermarket.

Saul, who had exomphalos major, is a happy, bright boy who loves his brother, his cat and everything to do with nature. A talented musician, he sings as a chorister.

Gilly, who had neonatal surgery for tetralogy of Fallot, is a busy toddler whose energy is not affected by her heart condition. She loves her sisters, singing and dancing – and bubbles.

Leo, who has a rare chromosomal microduplication, is healthy and happy, and learning to use a voice output device (a machine which converts typing to speech) to help him communicate. His fascination with washing machines continues.

Joel still hasn't decided whether he prefers the boomslang or the inland taipan.

*

In memory of Corey, Amber and Daisy.

Acknowledgements

Grateful thanks to:

Nina and Kris Hollington, without whose encouragement I would never have dared write this book, and Zoe Waxman, who turned things around at a crucial moment

Carole Tonkinson and Hockley Spare for their wise and kind editing, my meticulous copy-editor Jessica Cuthbert-Smith, Cindy Chan, Don Shanahan, Henry Lord, Jodie Mullish, Zainab Dawood and everyone else at Bluebird and Pan Macmillan

My smart agent Cathryn Summerhayes

The editors on newspapers, magazines and websites who first commissioned me to write on fetal and neonatal medicine and disability, with special thanks to Tamsin Kelly

All the staff at UCH, the Karolinska, GOSH, King's, CHOP, RasopathiesNet and other hospitals and scientific institutions who welcomed me to observe, checked facts and answered questions. Special thanks to my expert fact checkers: Anna David, Kay Davies, Martin Kostolny, Judith Meek and Charles Rodeck. And to my general medical fact checkers: Zoe Rooney and my father Siamon Gordon. Also thanks: Scott Adzick, Stuart Campbell, Kate Cross, Martin Elliott, Sian Harding, Holly Hedrick, Greg Heuer, Lori Howell, Mark Johnson, Giles Kendall, Gillian Kennedy, Siri Lilliesköld,

Neil Marlow, Joan Morris, Kypros Nicolaides, Pranav Pandya, Donald Peebles, Rebecca Proudfoot, Natalie Rintoul, Alex Robertson, Beth Stronach and Marco Tartaglia. And: Ashley Moore, Lisa Schoyer, Natalie Solimeo, Sharon Spiteri, Erica Stewart, ARC, Bliss, EUROCAT, SANDS

All the mothers and fathers who shared their experiences with me, including those I couldn't include in the book

The Society of Authors Authors' Foundation for their generous grant

Dr Caroline Dunn for intelligent interview transcriptions

The helpful staff at the Wellcome Unit for the History of Medicine Library, University of Oxford; Bodleian Library, University of Oxford; and the Wellcome Library, Wellcome Trust

Alan Schwarz and Steve Silberman for advice

My family of writers: my mother Lyndall Gordon and husband Philip Clark

And above all thanks to the NHS for giving me my children.

Notes on Sources

PREFACE

1   Ian Brown, *The Boy in the Moon*, Random House, 2009, pp95–6

ABNORMALITY

1   From a survey of the UK in 2012 we can say that around seven fetal medicine centres in England offered laser surgery for TTTS and around eighteen fetal medicine centres offered fetal blood transfusion. Author interview Anna David, November 2018

2   VM Crosse, *The Premature Baby*, J&A Churchill, reprinted 1946, p96

HIGH-RISK CASE

1   Michael Harrison, *Atlas of Fetal Surgery*, Chapman & Hall, 1996, p194

2   https://www.ucsf.edu/news/2011/02/9366/ucsf-surgeon-reflects-performing-worlds-first-fetal-surgery-30-years-ago, accessed 21 June 2018

3   https://surgicalinnovations.ucsf.edu/spotlight/innovator-profiles/michael-harrison,-md.aspx, accessed 21 June 2018

4   https://www.ucsf.edu/news/2011/02/9366/ucsf-surgeon-reflects-performing-worlds-first-fetal-surgery-30-years-ago, accessed 21 June 2018

5   Michael Harrison interview, *The First Foetal Surgery*, BBC World Service, 10 May 2018

6   Michael Harrison, 'Historical Perspective', in M Harrison et al. (eds), *The Unborn Patient: The Art and Science of Fetal Therapy*, Saunders, 2001

7   Author interview Charles Rodeck, 2017

8   Harrison, *Atlas of Fetal Surgery*, p12

9   https://surgicalinnovations.ucsf.edu/spotlight/innovator-profiles/michael-harrison,-md.aspx, accessed 21 June 2018

10   Harrison, 'Historical Perspective'

11   *Twice Born: Stories from the Special Delivery Unit*, PBS documentary, 2015

12   Harrison interview, *The First Foetal Surgery*

13   Author interview Lori Howell, 2018

14   Author interview Greg Heuer, 2018

15   Author interview Scott Adzick, 2018

16   Harrison interview, *The First Foetal Surgery*

17   https://surgicalinnovations.ucsf.edu/spotlight/innovator-profiles/michael-harrison,-md.aspx, accessed 21 June 2018

18   Harrison, *Atlas of Fetal Surgery*, p21

19   https://www.sfgate.com/health/article/SAN-FRANCISCO-First-foetal-surgery-survivor-2348923.php, accessed 21 June 2018

20   Harrison, *Atlas of Fetal Surgery*, p65

21   https://www.ncbi.nlm.nih.gov/pubmed/3724830 accessed 27 June 2018

22   Author interview Charles Rodeck

23   https://www.ncbi.nlm.nih.gov/pubmed/3724830, accessed 27 June 2018

24   Harrison, *Atlas of Fetal Surgery*, p210

25   Harrison, 'Historical Perspective'

26   Harrison, *Atlas of Fetal Surgery*, p19

27   Harrison, 'Historical Perspective'

28   Author interview Scott Adzick, 2018

29   Author interviews Stuart Campbell, Kypros Nicolaides and Charles Rodeck, 2017

30   Author interviews Stuart Campbell, Kypros Nicolaides and Charles Rodeck, 2017

31   Harrison, *Atlas of Fetal Surgery*, p194

32   Harrison, *Atlas of Fetal Surgery*, p126

33   http://www.uhs.nhs.uk/OurServices/Childhealth/Neonatalsurgery/Conditionswetreat/CongenitalDiaphragmaticHernia.aspx, accessed 10 July 2017

34 E Kirmisson, *A Handbook of the Surgery of Children*, Hodder & Stoughton, 1910, p93

35 https://www.ucsf.edu/news/2011/02/9366/ucsf-surgeon-reflects-performing-worlds-first-fetal-surgery-30-years-ago, accessed 21 June 2018

36 Author interview Kypros Nicolaides, 2017

37 Author interview Scott Adzick, 2018

38 Harrison, *Atlas of Fetal Surgery*, p126

39 Author interview Kypros Nicolaides, 2017

40 Harrison, *Atlas of Fetal Surgery*, p136

41 https://www.nhs.uk/conditions/spina-bifida, accessed 23 November 2018

42 Author interview Greg Heuer, 2018

43 Author interview Greg Heuer, 2018

44 Author interview Scott Adzick, 2018

45 Author interview Greg Heuer, 2018

46 https://ispdhome.org/ISPD/SIGs/Foetal_Therapy_Map.aspx, accessed 7 June 2018

47 Author interview Anna David, 2018

48 Laurie Scudder and N Scott Adzick, '20 Years in Fetal Surgery', Medscape.org, June 2015

STABS IN THE DARK

1 Harrison, 'Historical Perspective'

2 Karen Newman, *Fetal Positions*, Stanford University Press, 1996, p27

3 Newman, *Fetal Positions*, p33

4 Harrison, 'Historical Perspective'

5 Joanne Begiato, 'Breeding a Little Stranger: Managing Uncertainty in Pregnancy in Later Georgian England', in J Evans and C Meehan (eds), *Perceptions of Pregnancy from the Seventeenth to the Twentieth Century*, Palgrave Macmillan, 2017, p25

6 George Frederic Still, *The History of Paediatrics* (first published 1931), Dawsons, 1965, pp346–7

7 Newman, *Fetal Positions*, p58

8 Still, *The History of Paediatrics*, p347

9 Ann Dally, *Women under the Knife: A History of Surgery*, Castle, 1991, p134

10 Author interview Charles Rodeck, 2017

11   A. Susan Williams, *Women and Childbirth in the Twentieth Century*, Sutton Publishing, 1997, p101

12   Geoffrey Chamberlain, *From Witchcraft to Wisdom: A History of Obstetrics and Gynaecology in the British Isles*, Royal College of Obstetricians and Gynaecologists, 2007, p 176

13   https://www.nct.org.uk/pregnancy/rhesus-negative-blood-and-pregnancy, accessed 23 June 2017

14   Author interview Charles Rodeck, 2017

15   http://www.nytimes.com/2002/07/04/world/alice-stewart-95-linked-x-rays-to-diseases.html, 13 June 2017

16   S Campbell, 'Early Sonographic Prenatal Diagnosis', *Prenatal Diagnosis*, 30, 2010 and S Campbell, 'A Short History of Sonography in Obstetrics and Gynaecology', *Facts, Views and Vision in ObGyn*, 5(3), 2013

17   Author interview Stuart Campbell, 2017

18   Chamberlain, *From Witchcraft to Wisdom*, pp224, 225

19   EA Tansey and DA Christie (eds), *Looking at the Unborn: Historical Aspects of Obstetric Ultrasound*, Wellcome, 2000

20   Campbell, 'A Short History of Sonography in Obstetrics and Gynaecology'

21   Ian Donald, J MacVicar and TG Brown, 'Investigation of Abdominal Masses by Pulsed Ultrasound', *Lancet*, 7 June 1958, 1192–4

22   Campbell, 'Early Sonographic Prenatal Diagnosis'

23   Donald et al., 'Investigation of Abdominal Masses', 1191

24   Author interview Stuart Campbell, 2017

25   Author interview Stuart Campbell, 2017

26   Campbell, 'A Short History of Sonography in Obstetrics and Gynaecology'

27   Author interview Stuart Campbell, 2017

28   S Campbell, FD Johnstone, EM Holt, P May, 'Anencephaly: Early Ultrasonic Diagnosis and Active Management', *Lancet*, 9 December 1972

29   Chamberlain, *From Witchcraft to Wisdom*, p225

30   Author interview Stuart Campbell, 2017

31   Campbell et al., 'Anencephaly'

32   Campbell et al., 'Anencephaly'

33   Author interview Stuart Campbell, 2017

34   http://www.sites.hps.cam.ac.uk/visibleembryos/s7_4.html, accessed 14 June 2017 and Newman, *Fetal Positions*, pp10–11

35   https://en.wikipedia.org/wiki/Lennart_Nilsson, accessed 14 June 2017

36 Newman, *Fetal Positions*, p25

37 Monica J Casper, *The Making of the Unborn Patient: A Social Anatomy of Fetal Surgery*, Rutgers University Press, 1998, p66

38 Author interview Charles Rodeck, 2017

39 Author interview Charles Rodeck, 2017

40 Author interview Charles Rodeck, 2017

41 Author interview Charles Rodeck, 2017

42 Author interview Charles Rodeck, 2017

43 Author interview Pranav Pandya, 2018

BIRTH

1 Jeffrey P Baker, *The Machine in the Nursery*, Johns Hopkins University Press, 1996, p10

2 Baker, *The Machine in the Nursery*, p. 25 and Thomas Cone, *History of the Care and Feeding of the Premature Infant*, Lippincott Williams & Wilkins, 1985, Preface

3 Pierre Budin, *The Nursling*, Caxton, 1907, p9

4 PM Dunn, 'Perinatal Lessons from the Past: Stéphane Tarnier', *Archives of Disease in Childhood – Foetal and Neonatal Edition*, 86, 2002

5 Julius Hess, *Premature and Congenitally Diseased Infants*, J & A Churchill, 1923 p206

6 Budin, *The Nursling*, pp10–12

7 Budin, *The Nursling*, p3

8 Introduction by Alexander Simpson to Budin, *The Nursling*

9 http://www.bbc.co.uk/news/magazine-36321692, accessed 12 September 2017 (all information on Martin Couney from this article)

10 Hess, *Premature and Congenitally Diseased Infants*, pp230–1

11 Crosse, *The Premature Baby*, pp11–102

12 PM Dunn, 'Sir Leonard Parsons of Birmingham (1879–1950) and Antenatal Paediatrics', *Archives of Disease in Childhood – Foetal and Neonatal Edition*, 86, 2001, F66

13 Herbert Barrie quoted in DA Christie and EM Tansey (eds), *Origins of Neonatal Intensive Care. Wellcome Witnesses to Twentieth Century Medicine*, vol. 9, Wellcome Trust Centre for the History of Medicine at UCL, 2001

14 Baker, *The Machine in the Nursery*, p11

15 Herbert Barrie (and mentions of him on pages that follow) quoted in Christie and Tansey, *Origins of Neonatal Intensive Care*

16 Author interview Judith Meek, 2018

17 Neil McIntosh quoted in Christie and Tansey, *Origins of Neonatal Intensive Care*

18 Author interview Judith Meek, 2018

19 A 1964 paper from Toronto reported only one baby with RDS surviving after ventilation. At UCH, Os managed to reach a 30 per cent survival rate by the late 1960s. Professor Oswald Reynolds, quoted in Christie and Tansey, *Origins of Neonatal Intensive Care*

20 Christie and Tansey, *Origins of Neonatal Intensive Care*, p17

21 http://www.nytimes.com/2013/07/30/health/a-kennedy-babys-life-and-death.html, accessed 27 November 2017

22 HL Halliday, 'Surfactants: Past, Present and Future', *Journal of Perinatology*, May 2008

23 Christie and Tansey, *Origins of Neonatal Intensive Care*, pii

24 Peter Dunn quoted in Christie and Tansey, *Origins of Neonatal Intensive Care*

25 Christie and Tansey, *Origins of Neonatal Intensive Care*, pp49–55

26 Christie and Tansey, *Origins of Neonatal Intensive Care*, p56

27 Christie and Tansey, *Origins of Neonatal Intensive Care*, p39

28 https://councilfordisabledchildren.org.uk/news-opinion/news/numbers-children-complex-needs-50-2004, accessed 27 November 2017

29 Baby Doe story from C Everett Koop, *Koop: The Memoirs of America's Family Doctor*, Random House, 1991, pp240–59 and https://embryo.asu.edu/pages/baby-doe-rules-1984

30 Crosse, *The Premature Baby*, p138

31 Author interview with Neil Marlow, 2016

INTENSIVE CARE

1 Catherine Musemuche, *Small*, Dartmouth College Press, 2014, pp32–45

2 Christie and Tansey, *Origins of Neonatal Intensive Care*, p69

3 Pamela A Davies, 'Low Birthweight Infants: Immediate Feeding Recalled', *Archives of Disease in Childhood*, 66, 1991, pp551–3

4 Davies, 'Low Birthweight Infants'

5 Peter Dunn quoted in Christie and Tansey, *Origins of Neonatal Intensive Care*

6 Hess, *Premature and Congenitally Diseased Infants*, p168

DIAGNOSIS

1 Jacqueline Noonan, 'Hypertelorism with Turner Phenotype', *American Journal of Diseases in Childhood*, 1968

2 Interviews with Dr Noonan, Iowa Public Radio, February 2014 and Blogtalkradio.com, February 2010

3 Judith L Ross et al., 'Turner Syndrome: Toward Early Recognition and Improved Outcomes', Medscape.org, accessed 27 October 2017

4 JA Noonan, 'Noonan Syndrome: A Historical Perspective', *Heart Views*, 2002

5 Undiagnosed.org.uk, accessed 11 October 2017

6 https://ghr.nlm.nih.gov/gene/PTPN11#conditions, accessed 23 August 2018

7 Thanks to RasopathiesNet for this explanation

8 Psychopathological features in F Perrino et al., 'Noonan Syndrome', *European Journal of Paediatric Neurology*, 2017

9 There is some evidence older men can pass along this de novo mutation in their sperm. Author interview, Beth Stonach from RasopathiesNet, 2018

10 Marco Tartaglia et al., 'Mutations in PTPN11, Encoding the Protein Tyrosine Phosphatase SHP-2, Cause Noonan Syndrome', *Nature Genetics*, 2001

11 C Ruth Jamieson et al., 'Mapping a Gene for Noonan Syndrome to the Long Arm of Chromosome 12', *Nature Genetics*, 1994

12 William Tidyman and Katherine Rauen, 'The Rasopathies: Developmental Syndromes of the RAS/MAPK Pathway', *Current Opinions in Genetics and Development*, 2009

13 According to Pia Ostergaard, reader in Human Genetics, St George's Hospital

14 Donald Paterson, *Sick Children*, Cassell, 1956, pp396, 400

15 According to Paul Hunt, a researcher from Mencap

16 https://www.genome.gov/26524120/chromosomes-fact-sheet/, accessed 31 January 2018

17 https://library.down-syndrome.org/en-gb/research-practice/06/1/john-langdon-down-man-message, accessed 31 January 2018

18 Siddhartha Mukherjee, *The Gene: An Intimate History*, Bodley Head, 2016, p267

19   DA Christie and EM Tansey (eds) (2003) 'Genetic Testing', *Well-come Witnesses to Twentieth Century Medicine*, vol. 17, Wellcome Trust Centre for the History of Medicine at UCL, p20

20   Mukherjee, *The Gene*, p267

21   Carlo Valenti et al., 'Cytogenetic Diagnosis of Down's Syndrome in Utero', *Journal of the American Medical Association*, 207, 1969

22   Caroline Ogilvie, 'Cytogenics', in Rodeck and Whittle, *Foetal Medicine*, Churchill Livingstone Elsevier, 2009, pp305–9

23   Boaz Weisz and Charles Rodeck, 'Invasive Diagnostic Procedures', in Rodeck and Whittle, *Foetal Medicine*, pp292–5

24   J Haddow, G Palomaki, J Canick and G Knight, 'Prenatal Screening for Open Neural Tube Defects and Down's Syndrome', in Rodeck and Whittle, *Foetal Medicine*

25   Haddow et al., 'Prenatal Screening for Open Neural Tube Defects and Down's Syndrome'

26   Haddow et al., 'Prenatal Screening for Open Neural Tube Defects and Down's Syndrome' and https://www.telegraph.co.uk/news/health/news/6440705/Three-babies-aborted-every-day-due-to-Downs-syndrome.html, accessed 13 July 2018

27   Author interview Kypros Nicolaides, 2017

28   Author interview Pranav Pandya, 2018

29   Olav Lepaire et al., 'Non-Invasive Screening and Diagnosis from Maternal Blood', in Rodeck and Whittle, *Foetal Medicine*, p283

30   https://www.technologyreview.com/s/513691/prenatal-dna-sequencing, accessed 17 May 2018

31   National Congenital Anomaly and Rare Disease Registration Service (NCARDRS) figures 2014, reported by Sarah Stevens, Public Health Consultant, Registry lead, NCARDRS

32   https://www.cbsnews.com/news/down-syndrome-iceland, accessed 2 May 2018

33   https://www.gov.uk/government/uploads/system/uploads/attachment_data/file/652083/Abortion_stats_England_Wales_2016.pdf, accessed 31 January 2018

34   https://www.bpas.org/abortion-care/abortion-treatments/the-abortion-pill/feticide, accessed 13 July 2018

35   Margaret Wynn, *Prevention of Handicap and the Health of Women*, Routledge, 1979, pp12–13

36   https://www.downs-syndrome.org.uk/about/general/, accessed 6 February 2018

37 https://www.thecut.com/2017/11/raising-child-with-cystic-fibrosis.
html?_ga=2.177052709.1238175379.1547118530-812552985.150123
6218, accessed 13 January 2019

38 https://www.natera.com/press-releases/natera-inc-announces-
launch-vistara-single-gene-mutation-nipt, accessed 17 January 2018

39 https://www.mothercare.com/babybond.html, accessed 10 January
2019

40 https://www.nhs.uk/conditions/klinefelters-syndrome/, accessed 17
May 2018

41 https://www.technologyreview.com/s/513691/prenatal-dna-sequenc
ing, accessed 17 May 2018

'MUM'

1   Koop, *Koop: The Memoirs of America's Family Doctor*, p117

2   Budin, *The Nursling*, p68

3   Koop, *Koop: The Memoirs of America's Family Doctor*, p104

4   Budin, *The Nursling*, p13

5   Budin, *The Nursling*, p36

6   Budin, *The Nursling*, p36

7   Hess, *Premature and Congenitally Diseased Infants*, p126

8   Crosse, *The Premature Baby*, pp57–8

9   https://www.theatlantic.com/health/archive/2017/02/kangaroo-
care/515844/, accessed 11 April 2018

10 https://www.laleche.org.uk/meeting-needs-premature-babies-
kangaroo-mother-care/, accessed 11 January 2018

11 https://www.todaysparent.com/baby/newborn-care/preemie-care-
now-in-hands-of-parents, accessed 11 April 2018

12 Dally, *Women under the Knife*, Introduction

13 Newman, *Fetal Positions*, p51

14 Newman, *Fetal Positions*, p61

OPERATION

1   Kate Bull, *Open Hearts*, Elliott & Thompson, 2016, p215

2   Musemuche, *Small*, p11

3   Bull, *Open Hearts*, p175

4   Bull, *Open Hearts*, p32

5   https://www.achaheart.org/your-heart/health-information/tetra
logy-of-fallot, accessed 3 May 2018

6 Koop, *Koop: The Memoirs of America's Family Doctor*, p75
7 John G Raffensberger, *Children's Surgery: A Worldwide History*, McFarland & Co., 2012, p53
8 Raffensberger, *Children's Surgery*, p77
9 Koop, *Koop: The Memoirs of America's Family Doctor*, p76
10 Musemuche, *Small*, pp23–5
11 Details about Koop from Koop, *Koop: The Memoirs of America's Family Doctor*, pp76-117
12 Bull, *Open Hearts*, p174
13 Bull, *Open Hearts*, p99
14 Musemuche, *Small*, p18
15 Author interview Martin Elliott, 2017
16 Author interview Martin Elliott, 2017
17 Martin Elliott, 'The Size of a Walnut: Your Heart in their Hands', lecture, Gresham College, 25 May 2016
18 Bull, *Open Hearts* p130
19 Bull, *Open Hearts*, p22
20 E Kirmisson, *A Handbook of the Surgery of Children*, Hodder & Stoughton, 1910, p806
21 Author interview Alex Robertson, 2018

LATER

1 https://www.dailysignal.com/2014/12/09/elijahs-story-life-saved-birth, accessed 5 May 2018
2 https://www.thetimes.co.uk/article/my-nightmare-in-hospital-ptb9rnb6drk, accessed 28 March 2018
3 Author interview with Judith Meek, 2015
4 https://www.ncbi.nlm.nih.gov/pmc/articles/PMC3820298, accessed 5 May 2018
5 http://www.epicure.ac.uk/overview/main-challenges/, accessed 19 January 2019
6 https://www.telegraph.co.uk/news/science/science-news/12156081/Premature-babies-set-back-by-dungeon-incubators.html, accessed 5 May 2018
7 https://www.seminperinat.com/article/S0146-0005(16)30080-5/abstract?cc=y=, accessed 5 May 2018
8 http://www.sec-ed.co.uk/best-practice/the-emerging-new-sens-of-students-born-prematurely, accessed 5 May 2018

9   https://www.ncbi.nlm.nih.gov/pmc/articles/PMC3820298, accessed 5 May 2018

10 http://www.biomedcentral.com/1471-2431/13/25, accessed 5 May 2018

11 Author interview Neil Marlow, 2016

12 Alessandra Piontelli, *From Foetus to Child: An Observational and Psychoanalytic Study*, Routledge, 1992

13 Sigmund Freud, *Inhibitions, Symptoms and Anxiety* (first published 1925), in *Standard Edition of the Complete Psychological Works of Sigmund Freud, Vol. 20*, Vintage Classics, 2001, p138

14 Koop, *Koop: The Memoirs of America's Family Doctor*, p246

15 Stephanie Nimmo, *Was This in the Plan?*, Hashtag Press, 2017 and Stephanie Nimmo, *Goodbye Daisy*, Hashtag Press, 2018 and wasthisintheplan.co.uk

16 Author interview Mark Johnson, 2018

KNOWING

1   https://www.natera.com/press-releases/natera-inc-announces-launch-vistara-single-gene-mutation-nipt, accessed 17 January 2018

2   Brown, *The Boy in the Moon*, p75

3   https://www.theguardian.com/commentisfree/2017/jul/12/charlie-gard-doctors-speak-out-hospital-staff?CMP=fb_gu, accessed 13 July 2018

4   https://www.nejm.org/doi/pdf/10.1056/NEJM199612123352404, accessed 17 August 2018

5   Author interview Mark Johnson, 2018

6   https://www.npr.org/sections/health-shots/2017/06/21/532601431/survivors-of-childhood-diseases-struggle-to-find-care-as-adults, accessed May 2018